first place 4 health

member's guide

Published by Gospel Light
Ventura, California, U.S.A.
www.gospellight.com
Printed in the U.S.A.

Caution: The information contained in this book is intended to be solely for
informational and educational purposes. It is assumed that the First Place 4 Health
participant will consult a medical or health professional before beginning this or any
other weight-loss or physical fitness program.

Library of Congress Cataloging-in-Publication Data
First Place 4 Health member's guide / First Place 4 Health.
p. cm.
ISBN 978-0-8307-4524-1 (trade paper)
1. Spiritual life—Christianity. 2. Spiritual formation. 3. Health—Religious aspects—Christianity.
I. First Place 4 Health (Organization) II. Title: First Place for Health member's guide.
BV4501.3.F5695 2008
613.2—dc22

2008000346

1 2 3 4 5 6 7 8 9 10 / 15 14 13 12 11 10 09 08

Rights for publishing this book outside the U.S.A. or in non-English languages are administered
by Gospel Light Worldwide, an international not-for-profit ministry. For additional information,
please visit www.glww.org, email info@glww.org, or write to Gospel Light Worldwide,
1957 Eastman Avenue, Ventura, CA 93003, U.S.A.

contents

Section Four: Body

welcome to
first place 4 health!

Congratulations, and welcome to First Place 4 Health! By joining a First Place 4 Health group, you have taken an important step toward total health, wholeness and living a life that is pleasing to God. You have also become part of a worldwide fellowship of committed Christians who are seeking to bring balance and harmony to their lives. By keeping Christ first in all things and following the principles set forth in His Word, these men and women are striving to honor God in all aspects of their being. No matter what your diet and health history is, First Place 4 Health can herald the beginning of a new, healthier you. If you will commit yourself to the task at hand, give God and First Place 4 Health time to work in you, and wholeheartedly begin the process of making daily choices that support life and health, you *will* experience the First Place 4 Health miracle. You will have peace, purpose and a passion for God that you never dreamed possible. And, in the process, you will achieve your fitness and health goals.

When most people think about getting in shape, they immediately think about their body: maintaining the proper weight, living an active lifestyle, possessing flexibility and stamina, and remaining disease free. Certainly physical vitality is an important component of any health program. Caring for the physical body is an important part of the First Place 4 Health program, too. But Scripture makes clear that physical wellness is not the only area that impacts total health and well-being. When Jesus was asked by the religious leaders of His day which commandment was the most important, He declared, "Love the Lord your God with all your heart and with all your soul and with all your mind and with all your strength" (Mark 12:30). Humanity's greatest thoughts, highest reasoning and most creative imaginings fall far short of God's plan for our ultimate good as summed up in that God-breathed truth.

It has been said that God's kingdom is a paradoxical kingdom—an upside-down kingdom. God's way of thinking is different from our human thought process. In Isaiah 55:8, we read, "For my thoughts are not your thoughts, neither are your ways my ways, declares the LORD." Not only does God think different from how we think, but He also looks at things through different eyes: "The LORD does not look at the things man looks at. Man looks at the outward appearance, but the LORD looks at the heart" (1 Samuel 16:7). God is sovereign, supreme and all-knowing. Therefore, His thinking does not lack anything, and His eyes see the truth about each of us. Yet even though He knows all about us, God loves us with an unconditional love. We do not have to be perfect to earn the grace He freely gives us. And not only does God love us unconditionally, but our sovereign Lord is always active and working in our lives to bring about His glory and our highest good. What an awesome God we worship and serve!

God's plan for us is not only perfect, but it also goes far beyond what we could possibly envision. Throughout the pages of the Bible, our gracious God promises that if we trust Him completely—and seek Him more than we seek anything else on Earth—He will bring balance, healing and wholeness into every aspect of our life. That's a wonderful promise that we can claim when we are doing our part by ordering our lives according to God's good and perfect plan.

how has first place changed?

First Place began in 1981, when a God-given desire to establish a Christ-centered weight-control program was placed in the hearts of a group of committed Christians. Confident that God had called them to this important work, they began their pursuit with a basic premise: *Because God has saved us from our sins and given us an abundant life, why can't we, as Christians, use that same power in the area of weight control?*

With that question in mind, they began to develop a program that would meet the needs of Christian men and women who wanted to use solid biblical principles to bring the care of their physical bodies under the Lordship of Jesus Christ. It was an immense assignment; but knowing that God had called them to the task, these First Place pioneers placed all their hopes and aspirations in God and began the project. They prayed, studied and read; then they prayed some more; and as they began to write down what God had revealed to them, First Place began to take shape!

Through prayer and study, the First Place founders discerned that in order to be effective, this new program would need to include Scripture reading, prayer, Bible study, Scripture memory, small-group accountability and support, a proven commonsense nutrition plan, exercise and record keeping. They chose Matthew 6:33 as the plan's theme verse because they knew that keeping Christ first in their lives was the key to success in the program: "Seek first his kingdom and his righteousness, and all these things will be given to you as well." Since their aim was for growth in all areas of life—physical, mental, emotional and spiritual—they focused on Jesus' words in Mark 12:30: "Love the Lord your God with all your heart and with all your soul and with all your mind and with all your strength."

These core beliefs remain the foundation of the First Place 4 Health program today. We are convinced that we can only achieve balance in every area of life by putting our relationship with Jesus Christ first, not just in theory, but also in purposeful action that leads to positive transformation.

First Place has always had three underlying themes:

1 *Christ-centered priorities* (Bible study, prayer and Scripture memory)

2 *Choices for total health* (addressing the whole person—body, mind, emotions and spirit)

3 *Community* (support and accountability through small groups)

These three principles are still our core message!

Having made the decision to love God with all our heart, soul, mind and strength is just the beginning of the First Place 4 Health journey. The next step is to allow that all-important decision to manifest itself in the way we live our daily lives. That is why we added the words "4 Health" to the First Place name. We felt that it was important to clearly state that giving Christ first place is about healthy, balanced living that involves our body, our mind, our emotions and our spirit.

We have also simplified the program with new materials that have been reorganized for easy access. For example, the health topics for assigned reading (formerly called "wellness worksheets") used to be part of each individual Bible study. Now these same health topics will be contained in one book—*Simple Ideas for Healthy Living*. This will allow your group to read, discuss and benefit from the wisdom of these valuable worksheets no matter which Bible study you are currently working through. The original First Place Bible studies have been rewritten to give fresh meaning and application to the program's core memory verses. Our members kit now includes some exciting new DVDs that will add more depth and dimension to the time-honored First Place program. The all-new First Place 4 Health materials will help you make positive changes in your thought patterns and the way you handle your emotions, the way you nourish and recharge your body with food and exercise, and the way you relate to God, yourself and others. We've also provided a navigation sheet in the Member's Kit to explain how to use each of these tools for maximum benefit.

First Place has always taught—and will continue to teach—the basic disciplines named in the original nine commitments; for example, mental balance is found in renewing the mind through Scripture. But *the language and delivery of the message is different.* The emphasis now is on *acknowledging the preeminence of God* in all of life, *learning what Scripture says about how we are to live* and *making healthy choices for positive change to balance the four areas of life:*

1 Body (how we fuel and recharge ourselves)

2 Mind (our thought patterns and priorities)

3 Emotions (the quality of our relationship with self and others)

4 Spirit (our relationship with God through Jesus Christ)

your first place 4 health journey!

First Place has always been about a personal relationship with God, enhanced by group encouragement, support and accountability. Although we are individually accountable before God, He designed us to be in community. We were created to be dependent on God and interdependent on one another. Therefore, we are built up and strengthened in our faith as God's Holy Spirit works in and through our interaction with others in our group.

Now more than ever, your First Place 4 Health group will be a haven of support and encouragement as you move forward together. This circle of supportive friends will hold you accountable for the way you manage your First Place 4 Health program. Grace will be extended when you don't choose well, and encouragement will be given to get you back on track when you slip back into old patterns of behavior. Within your First Place 4 Health group, you will experience the unconditional support of those walking beside you on this journey to health and wholeness. Their love and encouragement will help you make *lasting changes* for total health.

Although weight management is most often our motivation for joining a First Place 4 Health group, the focus is not just on the body—or on the number on the scale. That's a crucial difference between First Place 4 Health and other weight-loss programs. By applying disciplines that affect the whole person—the body, the mind, the heart and the spirit—you will not only experience physical health but will also experience total health—health for life!

While there are no quick fixes when it comes to achieving the balanced life that God intends for you to live, if you will consistently make the small choices that lead to positive change, *you will succeed!* Your life will be transformed when you do the next right thing, whether that means using less added sugar, parking your car farther from your destination to get additional exercise, or opening your Bible to read it for the first time. Whether you are new to First Place 4 Health or an old-timer making the transition from First Place to the new First Place 4 Health program, patience with the process is the pathway to success: patience with God, patience with self, and patience with those who share your First Place 4 Health journey.

It is vital that you accept yourself as you are and then allow God to move you toward health and wholeness in His good time. Inner healing must often come before the number on the scale begins to go down. God knows exactly what you need and is the One directing your First Place 4 Health program.

Our all-powerful God could certainly transform our body, mind, heart and spirit in the twinkling of an eye, should He choose to do so. However, our sovereign Lord is more interested in building mature Christian character than in obtaining instant results. "With the Lord a day is like a thousand years, and a thousand years are like a day" (2 Peter 3:8). Our transformation process begins the moment we accept Jesus Christ as our Lord and Savior and continues until we are taken up in glory to live with the Lord forever. This ongoing, lifelong journey is called sanctification: We are being renewed moment by moment, day by day, as we walk in sync with the Spirit and discern God's will and way for our life.

Even though our human mind and heart have been conditioned by the instant-makeover mentality of the society we live in, health and healing in God's kingdom are about process, and process takes time. Esther entered a one-year period of beauty treatments before being brought before King Xerxes (see Esther 2:12); Daniel and his companions began a three-year training process in preparation for serving King Nebuchadnezzar (see Daniel 1:5); the disciples went through an intense three-year internship before being commissioned to proclaim the good news of the Gospel of God's grace.

Through First Place 4 Health, we, too, are asked to enter a time of preparation as we grow in grace and knowledge and develop a body, mind, heart and spirit fit for the King's service. That's why you are asked to make a one-year commitment to the First Place 4 Health program rather than view this life-transforming program as a last-ditch effort, something to halfheartedly try before taking drastic measures that promise rapid results but do not promote total health. In the depths of your being, you promise yourself and God one year of wholehearted participation in First Place 4 Health so that through this program, God can transform you according to His great plan and purpose for your life.

Putting God first is the heart of the First Place 4 Health program. This Bible-centered precept has the power to bring fundamental life change as you seek to know God and do His revealed will. When you first joined First Place 4 Health, you became aware of the importance of keeping Christ first in all things. As you begin to incorporate the principles of First Place 4 Health into your life, you will take another step and then another in God's direction. Each new day will present you with new challenges and invite you to reaffirm your desire to honor God by practicing balanced self-care. As you keep walking on the path God has marked out for you, your life will begin to change in ways that you had only hoped for in the past.

Over time, what began with an acknowledgment of who God is and His right of first place in your thoughts, affections and day-to-day decisions will shift into a full-on pursuit of Him. Before long, you will know His ways and experience His power in place of your weaknesses. You will begin to express an ever-increasing gratefulness for His presence in all areas of your life. The more you surrender control to your Creator-God, the more fully you will find freedom from the bondage of negative thought patterns and behaviors. Paradoxically, victory comes through surrender, not through stubborn self-will. "'Not by might nor by power, but by my Spirit,' says the LORD Almighty" (Zechariah 4:6). This is opposite world thinking, but it *is* Kingdom thinking!

When you begin the First Place 4 Health journey, you may only notice small, subtle shifts in your priorities. However, as you begin to bring all areas of your life under the direction of your loving and compassionate Lord—the One who wants to free you from addictions, undesirable behaviors and negative emotions—positive change is guaranteed. You will find that getting in good physical shape will no longer hold first-place position when you define the things that constitute health. By God's grace, you will begin to realize that you are living for the One who created you and knows you best, the One whose truth will set you free. Before long you will find greater satisfaction in your internal changes than in seeing the needle of the weight scale move to the left! When your attitudes and behaviors begin to shift, not only will you experience physical freedom, but you also will no longer see weight loss as the most important achievement in your journey toward health. One day you will suddenly realize that your chief desire is to put God in the position of primary importance in all of your decisions. Decision by decision, day by day, you will have allowed God to become your chief counselor—and you will be confident that He will never steer you wrong. Restoration is a precious gift from God. Because of our Lord's mercy, compassion and love, each day is a new beginning in First Place 4 Health.

Although God's kingdom is an upside-down kingdom, it is not a disorderly kingdom. Our God is a God of decency and order. Built into His creation are specific spiritual principles, or laws, that are as real as the law of gravity is in the physical realm. Knowing God's spiritual kingdom principles will allow you to walk in sync with God's Spirit and benefit from the power these principles contain. Although there are many spiritual principles in God's universe, certain kingdom principles are especially important to your First Place 4 Health efforts:

- **Sowing and reaping.** The law of cause and effect is a basic tenet of life. In the Bible, this law is better known as sowing and reaping. "Do not be deceived: God cannot be mocked. A man reaps what he sows" (Galatians 6:7). "Whoever sows sparingly will reap sparingly, and whoever sows generously will also reap generously" (2 Corinthians 9:6). Elsewhere Scripture tells us that God "rewards those who earnestly seek him" (Hebrews 11:6). First Place 4 Health will yield abundant rewards in all four aspects of our life, provided we are willing to do our part in terms of human effort. When we put God first in all things and seek His kingdom and a right relationship with Him, we will be given all things. Conversely, the book of Proverbs gives us the whimsical example of the sluggard—the lazy one—who looks for a crop at harvest time but finds only weeds because he failed to till, plant and cultivate his land (see Proverbs 20:4; 24:30-31). Likewise, we cannot expect to reap First Place 4 Health benefits if we are not willing to do the work.

- **Replacing bad with good.** In Matthew 12:43-45, Jesus told about a man who cleaned his house but did not replace the bad with good. As a result, the evil spirit came back—bringing seven friends—and left the condition of the house worse than it was before the housecleaning began. As we eliminate the destructive behaviors that characterized our life prior to First Place 4 Health, it is important that we immediately replace them with life-affirming practices. We nourish what is good and weed out what is bad. This practice is often called weeding and feeding, or pulling weeds and planting flowers. Fleeing from the devil and drawing near to God is an excellent example of the principle of replacement (see James 4:7-8).

- **Taking personal responsibility.** Jesus told a parable about five wise bridesmaids and five foolish ones who were waiting for the bridegroom to appear (see Matthew 25:1-13). The five wise bridesmaids took oil for their lamps; the five foolish ones did not. When the bridegroom finally appeared, the foolish bridesmaids wanted to borrow oil from those who had been wise enough to bring extra, but they were not allowed to do so. What Jesus taught in this parable is that we are each personally responsible for maintaining a right relationship with Christ by keeping Him first in all things. When we join First Place 4 Health, we are indeed part of a group, but each of us is individually accountable to the Master. One First Place 4 Health group member cannot do the work God has called the others in the group to do, no matter how valiant his or her efforts.

First Place 4 Health is not about acquiring more head knowledge; it is about applying heart knowledge in practical ways that produce positive change. Most of us come to First Place 4 Health with enough factual information to create our own diet and exercise program. What we lack is heart knowledge, knowledge that has filtered down to the core of our being through daily application. Information that does not lead to transformation is not our goal in First Place 4 Health. Our goal is empowerment to make life-altering change: "For the kingdom of God is not a matter of talk but of power" (1 Corinthians 4:20).

Throughout *First Place 4 Health Member's Guide,* you will be asked to "Learn It" and then "Live It." Your responsibility is to take the information to heart so that the Holy Spirit can apply this life-changing program to the areas of your life that need revival. God has not given you "a spirit of timidity, but a spirit of power, of love and of self-discipline" (2 Timothy 1:7). As you take the action steps suggested by the First Place 4 Health material, God's power will begin to work in and through you. Step by step, choice by choice, your life will be transformed. The path will grow brighter every day because you are taking action rather than simply gathering facts.

Are you ready to choose the path of loving God with all your heart, soul, mind and strength? Just as soon as you take the first step, God will meet you and lead you the rest of the way. Our prayers are with you as you begin this exciting adventure. May God always have first place in your life!

the four-sided person

Love the Lord your God with all your heart and with all your soul
and with all your mind and with all your strength.

MARK 12:30

S oon after coming into First Place 4 Health, we begin to realize that our eating is not the only part of our life that is out of control. We soon discover that we are people who lack balance and harmony in many other areas of our life, too. By using the following illustration of a four-sided person, we can easily determine which areas of our life need the most attention. (Most of us have one strong area, one weak area, and two that are somewhere in between.)

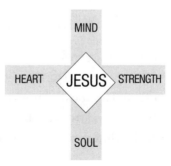

As you begin this exercise, carefully read the explanation of each of the four aspects of our being, which are listed below. Then study the crossed bars with the diamond at the center in the illustration of the four-sided person. Consider each area with regard to your current situation.

Begin by asking yourself the most important question, *Is Jesus really at the center of my life—is He both my Savior and my Lord?* If you can answer that question in the affirmative, completely color in the diamond at the center of the illustration. If Jesus is at the center in some but not all of the areas of your life, fill in the diamond-shaped area of the illustration appropriately. Realize that you cannot achieve balance in the other areas until you have placed yourself completely under the Lordship of Christ, and doing so needs to be your first priority.

Next, turn your attention to the four bars that represent your heart, soul, mind and strength. How much balance do you currently have in each of those aspects of your life? Indicate the amount of health and wholeness you're currently experiencing in each of those areas by shading in a corresponding portion of each bar. You might want to use a different colored pencil for each section.

Which bar contains the least amount of shading, and why do you think that is so? That's the area of your life that needs attention today. Do you see a pattern emerging between the balance and harmony you are experiencing and the degree to which you have surrendered your life to Christ? Remember, no matter how strong you may be in one area, you are only as strong as your weakest point!

No matter how lopsided, or empty, your chart looks right now, do not despair. You will find help to address the areas of your life that need attention within this member's guide. As you (1) apply yourself to the First Place 4 Health program, (2) begin to study God's Word, (3) interact with the others in your group, and (4) follow a prudent plan of eating and exercise, you will be simultaneously working to bring health and wholeness to all four areas of your being. Although the components are separate, they are also interrelated. Any action you take to bring health and wholeness in one area also brings healing to the other three. That's good news. It means that you're making progress and are able to address each place that needs God's healing touch as you concentrate on keeping Christ in first place.

EMOTIONAL HEALTH: "WITH ALL YOUR HEART"

To love God with all your heart includes the experience of genuine community—the fellowship of believers—and mutual encouragement. The emotional component also addresses your ability to handle the stresses of life. The apostle James compares the emotionally unstable person to a ship that is being tossed to and fro on a stormy sea (see James 1:6-8). The First Place 4 Health life plan for emotional wellness includes a weekly group meeting specifically designed to do several things:

- Combat your isolation
- Increase your optimism regarding personal change
- Provide you with information regarding effective coping techniques
- Promote the truth that you are loved by God
- Change your self-focus to a God-focus
- Provide you with a loving First Place 4 Health family of friends

- Build healthy interpersonal relationships for yourself rather than focus on a destructive relationship with food

Developing healthy interpersonal relationships begins by attending your First Place 4 Health meeting and by encouraging others. That is why these two activities are such an important part of your First Place 4 Health endeavors. The more successful you are in attendance and encouragement, the more successful you will be in the other areas of the First Place 4 Health program, too. Ecclesiastes 4:12 says, "Though one may be overpowered, two can defend themselves." You will be asked to reach out to other members of your First Place 4 Health group with intentional acts of encouragement. You will also learn to accept love and encouragement from them, which for many is a new behavior. It is often easier to give than to receive when it comes to emotional support, but healthy relationships require that we do both.

God wants us to love Him with our whole heart and to love others because He loves them, too. There is no better example of someone with emotional balance than Jesus. He cried when His friend Lazarus died; He had compassion for the sick and suffering; He got angry when the moneychangers defiled His Father's house. Galatians 5:22-23 names the fruit of the Spirit—"love, joy, peace, patience, kindness, goodness, faithfulness, gentleness and self-control"—and Jesus was all these values wrapped in human flesh. Although our Savior was a man of strong emotions, it was His Father's will, not His human emotions, that dictated His behavior. As you are changed into His likeness and image, that same emotional self-control can be yours! Emotional wellness will be one of the greatest benefits you enjoy from learning what it means to give Christ first place in this area of your life.

SPIRITUAL HEALTH: "WITH ALL YOUR SOUL"

Learning to love the Lord your God with all of your soul entails developing a personal, interactive relationship with the Lord Jesus Christ. Many of us who come to First Place 4 Health have participated in the Church for years, yet we have never developed an intimate relationship with our Lord and Master. The First Place 4 Health spiritual plan will teach you to spend time with the Lord on a daily basis in several ways:

- **Bible study.** The First Place 4 Health Bible studies are specifically written to help you apply the truth of God's Word to your life in practical ways that encourage health and fitness.

- **Scripture reading.** Daily scripture reading will expose you to the truth of God's Word. According to John 8:32, Jesus said, "You will know the truth, and the truth will set you free." God will speak to your heart as the Holy Spirit reveals God's truth to you and reminds you of Jesus' teaching.

● **Prayer.** Prayer is your time of daily conversation with God. You can remember how to come to God in prayer by using the acrostic F.I.R.S.T.:

Focus

Invite

Reconcile

Surrender

Trust

Once again, Jesus is our example when it comes to loving God with all our spirit. Even after ministering to the needs of the crowd well into the night, Jesus got up early in the morning to spend quiet time with His Father in heaven. After Jesus and His disciples had spent a long, tiring day tending to the needs of the sick and the crippled and the blind, Jesus asked the disciples to come away with Him to a quiet place to rest. Before each major decision in His ministry, Jesus prayed. When He was in agony in the Garden of Gethsemane, Jesus sought the will of His Father. By following our Savior's example, we can enjoy the peace of God that passes all understanding, no matter what circumstances we are in at the present moment (see Philippians 4:7). Spiritual health is vital to balance and harmony.

MENTAL HEALTH: "WITH ALL YOUR MIND"

Loving God with all your mind means that you let Him take every thought captive, especially those negative voices that keep you in doubt and despair. This will mean that you have to learn a new way of thinking. The battle for wellness starts in the mind. The Bible says that God's Word is a divine weapon, given to us so that we can overcome mental strongholds and renew and transform our mind so that we actually begin "to will and to act according to [God's] good purpose" (Philippians 2:13). The Bible tells us in 2 Corinthians 10:5 that we can "demolish arguments and every pretension that sets itself up against the knowledge of God, and we take captive every thought to make it obedient to Christ." The apostle Peter tells us that he wrote his epistle to stimulate us to "wholesome thinking" (2 Peter 3:1).

You will be asked to memorize one Scripture passage every week. Scripture memory will be a key element in learning to be obedient to all that God is asking you to do. Scripture memory will accomplish several things:

- Empower you to resist temptation
- Keep you on course as you move toward your First Place 4 Health goals
- Enable you to meditate on God's Word rather than give in to negative thinking
- Allow the Holy Spirit to bring to your mind at just the right time the verses you have stored in your heart

The book of Hebrews instructs us to "fix our eyes on Jesus, the author and perfecter of our faith" (Hebrews 12:2). When Jesus was tempted in the desert wilderness, His first and only defense was the "it is written" Word of God. At the beginning of His earthly ministry, Jesus read from the prophet Isaiah. While dying on the cross, Jesus quoted the first verse of Psalm 22. Scripture memory allowed Jesus to give glory to His Father in all circumstances. It will do the same for you.

As your mind is renewed, you will begin to develop the mind of Christ. This will allow you to accomplish certain goals:

- **Overcome anxiety about your present circumstances and your future destiny.** "Do not be anxious about anything, but in everything, by prayer and petition, with thanksgiving, present your requests to God" (Philippians 4:6).

- **Discern God's will.** "Then you will be able to test and approve what God's will is—his good, pleasing and perfect will" (Romans 12:3).

- **Have inseparable faith and obedience.** "It is God who works in you to will and act according to his good purpose" (Philippians 2:13).

This is a very impressive list of essential elements that will help you defeat the negative thinking that threatens to keep you in defeat and despair!

Another important aspect of loving God with all your mind is developing mindfulness. All positive change begins with awareness—and awareness requires accurate record keeping. Each day you will be asked to record your progress using a tool called the Live It Tracker. This written record will keep you from falling into vagueness or denial regarding your level of participation in the First Place 4 Health program. You will be able to live purposefully as you take the next right step toward your First Place 4 Health fitness goals. Mindfulness will also allow you to monitor your progress and evaluate your daily choices.

PHYSICAL HEALTH: "WITH ALL YOUR STRENGTH"

A lifestyle of physical health includes eating healthy foods, making time to exercise, getting enough rest, and learning how to enjoy quality recreation. This will not happen overnight, but you can make progress through your daily choices. You are living in the only physical body you will ever have on this earth, and Scripture tells us that care of our body is both an act of stewardship (see Romans 12:1) and a way of honoring God who dwells with us through the Holy Spirit (see 1 Corinthians 6:19).

You will care for your physical self primarily by exercising daily; eating well, which includes choosing quality foods in appropriate quantities; and balancing work, rest, relationships and recreation.

It is easy to look at the man Jesus and forget that while He was fully divine, He was also fully human. As He grew, Jesus worked as a carpenter. After He began His ministry, Jesus often experienced hunger and thirst, and He took time to rest as He walked the dusty roads of Galilee—probably traveling many miles each day on foot. After one particularly long day of healing and teaching, He was so tired that He went to sleep in the back of a boat on a stormy sea. He stumbled three times under the weight of the cross He carried to His own crucifixion. So Jesus understands our physical weaknesses and limitations and asks that we care for our physical body so that we can be His hands and feet, eyes and ears, voice and heart in a world still in need of His compassion and love.

Spirit

LEARN IT

- To know God requires that you establish a relationship with Him.
- Those who earnestly seek God will find Him.
- Keep Christ F.I.R.S.T. in your prayers.
- Change starts when you begin to infuse truth in your life. (It is God who is the ultimate source of truth, and it is His Word that tells you the most about truth.)
- There is a difference between reading Scripture and studying Scripture.
- Learn how to share your faith with others.
- How to become a Christian

LIVE IT

- Weight-loss begins on your knees.
- Create a quiet space and place to encounter God.
- Surrender your life to God each day with a simple prayer: *God, this day is for You.*
- Read your Bible daily, but dig deeper as well—*study* is different from *reading.*
- Record your spiritual journey and keep a thankfulness journal.
- Write your personal faith story.
- Accept Christ as your Lord and Savior.

getting to know God!

Be still, and know that I am God;
I will be exalted among the nations, I will be exalted in the earth.

PSALM 46:10

When most of us envision what being in relationship with God means, we immediately think of *doing*: what God can do for us and what we can do for Him. However, God's vision of what our relationship with Him is supposed to look like centers around *being*:

- Being still and knowing that He is God
- Being willing to sit at His feet and learn from Him
- Being nourished by His Word
- Being in daily conversation with Him
- Being grateful for the good things He has given us
- Being content with His abundant provision
- Being obedient to His revealed will
- Being surrendered to His plan and purpose for our life

Although salvation is a free gift from God, something we cannot work for or earn, we are each called to work out our salvation once we have been saved by God's grace. Much as we must exercise our physical bodies to build strength, stamina, flexibility and endurance, we must also exercise our spiritual muscles to "grow in the grace and knowledge of our Lord and Savior Jesus Christ" (2 Peter 3:18). How do we exercise our spiritual muscles? By spending quality time in God's presence, by speaking to Him in prayer and by meditating on His Word so that He can speak to us, too.

Throughout the First Place 4 Health material, you will read about the importance of spending quality time with God. We call it quiet time—our time alone with God, our opportunity to sit at the Master's feet and learn from Him. It is easy to understand the importance of spending time with the object of our affection on a human level. All we need to do is observe young lovers, regardless of their chronological age, to comprehend what getting to know another person on an intimate level involves: They talk together on the phone, write notes and letters, spend every possible moment together, discussing trivial things that suddenly have great importance because they are being shared with an important other. Yet most of us have a difficult time transferring that image to our relationship with God. Even those who have attended a church since childhood have not been taught the importance of developing an intimate, interactive relationship with God. And those of us who do know that we should spend time with God have no idea how to go about putting that concept into practice. It is one thing to talk about spending time with God but another to really do it!

establishing a quiet time!

Like all other components of the First Place 4 Health program, developing a live relationship with God is not a random act. We must intentionally seek God if we are to find Him! It's not that God plays Hide-and-Seek with us. He is always available to us; He invites us to come boldly into His presence; He reveals Himself to us in the pages of the Bible. And once we decide to earnestly seek Him, we are sure to find Him! When we delight in Him, our gracious God will give us the desires of our heart.

Spending time getting to know God involves four basic elements: a priority, a plan, a place and practice.

A PRIORITY

You can successfully establish a quiet time with God by making this meeting a daily priority. For most of us, that requires carving out time in our day so that we have time and space for this new relationship we are cultivating. Often this will mean less important things must be eliminated so that we will have time and space to meet with God. When speaking about Jesus, John the Baptist said, "He must become greater; I must become less" (John 3:30). You will undoubtedly find that to be true, too.

What might you need to eliminate from your current schedule so that spending quality time with God can become a priority?

A PLAN

Having made quiet time a priority, you will want to come up with a plan. This plan will include the time you have set aside to spend with God, and a general outline of how you spend your time in God's presence. Elements you should consider incorporating into your quiet time include the following:

- Singing a song of praise
- Reading a daily selection in a devotional book or reading a psalm
- Using a systematic Scripture reading plan so that you will be exposed to the whole truth of God's Word
- Completing your First Place 4 Health Bible study for that day
- Praying—silent, spoken and written prayer
- Writing in your spiritual journal

You will also want to make a list of the materials you will need to make your encounter with God more meaningful:

- A Bible
- Your First Place 4 Health Bible study
- Your prayer journal
- A pen and/or pencil
- A devotional book
- A Bible concordance

- A college-level dictionary
- A tape or CD player if music and praise songs will be part of your quiet time
- A box of tissues (Tears—both of sadness and joy—are often part of our quiet time with God!)

Think of how you would plan an important business meeting or social event, and then transfer that knowledge to your meeting time with God.

A PLACE

Having formulated a meeting-with-God plan, next you will need to create a meeting-with-God place. Of course, God is always with us; however, in order to have quality devotional time with Him, it is desirable that you find a comfortable meeting place. You will want to select a spot that is quiet and as distraction-free as possible. Being in the same place on a regular basis will help you remember what you are there for: to have an encounter with the true and living God! Having selected the place, put the materials you have determined to use in your quiet time into a basket or on a nearby table or shelf.

Take the time to establish your personal quiet time with God now. Tailor your quiet time to fit your needs—and the time you have allotted to spend with God. Although many people elect to meet with God early in the morning, for others afternoon or evening is best. There is no hard and fast rule about when your quiet time should be. The only essential thing is that you establish a quiet time! Start with a small amount of time that you know you can devote yourself to daily; you can be confident that as you consistently spend time with God each day, the amount of time you can spend will increase as you are ready for the next level of your walk with God.

I will meet with God from _____ to _____ daily.

I plan to use that time with God to _____

_____

Supplies I will need to assemble include _____

_____

My meeting place with God will be _____

PRACTICE

After you have chosen the time and place to meet God daily and you have assembled your supplies, there are four easy steps for a fruitful and worshipful time with the Lord.

Step 1: Clear Your Heart and Mind

"Be still, and know that I am God" (Psalm 46:10). Begin your quiet time by reading the daily Bible selection from a devotional guide or a psalm. If you are new in your Christian walk, *Streams in the Desert* by L. B. Cowman is an excellent devotional guide to start with. More mature Christians might benefit from *My Utmost for His Highest* by Oswald Chambers. Of course, you can use any devotional that has a strong emphasis on Scripture and prayer. (We have included more choices in the "First Place 4 Health Recommended Resources" in the back of this member's guide.)

Step 2: Read and Interact with Scripture

"I have hidden your word in my heart that I might not sin against you" (Psalm 119:11). As you open your Bible to read Scripture, ask the Holy Spirit to reveal something He knows that you need for this day through the reading of His Word. Always try to find a nugget to encourage or direct you through the day. As you read the Scripture passage, pay special attention to the words and phrases the Holy Spirit brings to your attention. Some words may seem to resonate in your soul. You will want to spend time meditating on the passage, asking God what lesson He is teaching you. After reading the Scripture passage over several times, ask yourself the following questions:

1. *In light of what I have read today, is there something I must now do? (**Confess a sin? Claim a promise? Follow an example? Obey a command? Avoid a situation?**)*

2. *How should I respond to what I've read today?*

Step 3: Pray

"Be clear minded and self-controlled so that you can pray" (1 Peter 4:7). Spend time conversing with the Lord in prayer. Prayer is such an important part of First Place 4 Health that there is an entire section in this member's guide devoted to the practice of prayer.

Step 4: Praise

"Praise the LORD, O my soul, and forget not all his benefits" (Psalm 103:2). End your quiet time with a time of praise. Be sure to thank the Lord of heaven and Earth for choosing to spend time with you!

Lord, teach us to pray!

Be joyful always; pray continually; give thanks in all circumstances,
for this is God's will for you in Christ Jesus.

1 THESSALONIANS 5:16-18

First Place 4 Health is founded on the principle of seeking God before anything else, and prayer is one of the best ways to spend time with Him. Prayer gives us access to the Creator of the universe! God loves us so much that He gave us prayer as a way to personally communicate with Him, and He with us. We pray, not only because we need and want to, but also because God desires communion with us. God created us to love Him and enjoy being in relationship with Him forever!

PRAYER JOURNAL

One of the best ways to carve out consistent time for prayer and to stay focused is to keep a prayer journal. Use your journal to write out your prayers. Keeping a prayer journal is also a great way to watch God answer your prayers—even when you don't realize why you're praying for a certain person or thing.

PRIVATE PRAYER

You are encouraged to converse with God each day in a way that fits your personality and lifestyle. Trust that God is interested in spending time with you, and He will help you find the time to pray if you will just allow Him to do so. If prayer is new to you, try using the F.I.R.S.T. method of prayer. The F.I.R.S.T. guide for your daily prayer time with God is only a suggestion. It is not the only way to pray, but it gives you an easy way to remember some of the important aspects of prayer. Let's take a look at each of the aspects in the F.I.R.S.T method.

F—Focus

It's easier to focus if you have a regular place where you meet with God each day. Find an isolated spot somewhere out of the main traffic area of your home or office so that you will not be interrupted or easily distracted. Keep nearby the supplies you have assembled. Using the same spot each day will help you focus on why you are there and ingrain the habit of spending time with God.

I—Invite

Once you are in your quiet place ready to meet with God, invite Him to join you there. You can do this by singing a praise song or hymn, or if you prefer, write the words of the song or a praise psalm from your Bible in your prayer journal. The purpose of this activity is to take the focus off of you and put it on the greatness of God.

A good beginning place is adoration. "Adoration" simply means praising God for who He is. When you begin your time of prayer, start by praising God for His character, for everything He is and for everything He has done. This might feel awkward to you at first; but with a little practice, you will find that praising God will elevate your mind to the right attitude for prayer.

The Lord's Prayer begins with adoration. Many of us learned this prayer when we were young. It's found in Matthew 6 (verses 9-13) and Luke 11 (verses 2-4). In Matthew, it begins: "Our Father in heaven, hallowed be your name." The word "hallowed" means sacred, honored or blessed. When we say that God's name is hallowed, we are showing that we adore Him.

R—Reconcile

Reconcile yourself with God; get into agreement with God and restore your harmonious relationship; agree with God that your sin is grievous in His sight. David stated this eloquently in Psalm 32:5: "Then I acknowledged my sin to you and did not cover up my iniquity. I said, 'I will confess my transgressions to the LORD'—and you forgave the guilt of my sin." In the New Testament, the apostle John said the same thing in 1 John 1:9: "If we confess our sins, he is faithful and just and will forgive us our sins and purify us from all unrighteousness."

After asking God to reveal anything you might have done or said in the last 24 hours that wasn't right and that you need to be aware of, sit quietly before Him. Ask Him to also show you where and when you neglected to do or say something that was right and would have been helpful to you or to someone else. Paul said it best in Romans 7:15: "I do not understand what I do. For what I want to do I do not do, but what I hate I do."

After the Holy Spirit reveals any wrong action, attitude of the heart and/or any words or good deeds that you could have said or done but didn't, tell God that you're sorry and ask

His forgiveness as well as His help in this area. If your sin involved another person, see if you can arrange a time to talk to the person and ask for his or her forgiveness before you next meet with God. Reconciling with God and with others keeps us clean and right with God and with other people.

S—Surrender

According to John 8:31-32, Jesus said, "If you hold to my teaching, you are really my disciples. Then you will know the truth, and the truth will set you free." Studying the Bible teaches you about God and what He desires for your life. Every word of the Bible is true, and as we study it, we begin to replace distorted thinking with the truth. Yet just knowing the truth is not enough. We must surrender to that truth; we must yield our stubborn self-will to God's will as revealed in the pages of the Bible. Surrender is best summed up in Jesus' words "Father . . . not my will, but yours be done" (Luke 22:42). You may find yourself surrendering the same issues over and over again until you are finally ready to yield yourself to God's will and be obedient to His teaching. When it comes to surrender, progress, not perfection, is our daily goal.

T—Trust

Finish your prayer time each day by placing your life and daily activities into God's loving hands. Proverbs 3:5-6 is a great passage about trust: "Trust in the LORD with all your heart and lean not on your own understanding; in all your ways acknowledge him, and he will make your paths straight." When we trust God, we acknowledge that we want His schedule to be our schedule. We say that if He wants to intervene in the plans we have made today, it is perfectly all right, because we trust Him to accomplish what He desires for us.

CORPORATE PRAYER

You will encounter another way to pray at a First Place 4 Health meeting. We believe in the importance of praying together as a group, so we pray at the beginning and at the end of every meeting. The prayer time at the beginning is usually short: Often it's simply to commit the meeting to the Lord and ask Him to help us focus on the material at hand. The prayer time at the end of each meeting usually lasts about 15 minutes. During this time, participants ask for prayer for themselves or for needs that affect their success in the program. (We encourage people to limit prayer requests to personal needs.)

As you make yourself vulnerable enough to ask for prayer for specific needs, you will see the mighty power of prayer at work. It is important to emphasize that prayer requests made during corporate prayer need to stay inside the group. We ask each participant to never share a prayer request with anyone outside the group. As a result, the members of the group know that their requests will remain confidential. When we have a safe place for our prayer requests, we can voice our deep concerns and anxieties—and they cease to have power over us.

Your First Place 4 Health Bible studies contain two prayer sheets. One is the Group Prayer Requests form at the end of each week. On it you can record any prayer requests from the members of your group and also check back to record the results of answered prayer. This prayer sheet remains in your Bible study.

The second form is also found at the end of each week in your Bible study (see also the following page), but this form is for your personal prayer request(s) unvoiced during the meeting. Typically, you and the other members of your group will fill out this form before each weekly meeting and place your sheets in a basket to be passed around for everyone to take one. The author of the prayer sheet you choose is the person you will pray for and encourage throughout the week. This is a great way to give and receive encouragement and support!

First Place 4 Health
Prayer Partner Form

4health

Date _____

Name _____

Home Phone (_____) _____

Work Phone (_____) _____

Email _____

Personal Prayer Concerns:

_____

_____

_____

_____

_____

_____

_____

_____

_____

_____

This form is for prayer requests that are personal to you and your journey in First Place 4 Health. Please complete this form and have it ready to turn in each week when you arrive at your group meeting.

prayer journaling: a personal testimony

by Carole Lewis

Believing that God wants His children to pray, I began writing my prayers in April 1990. For several years, I had resisted praying in this manner. Being a fun-loving individual, I felt that writing my prayers would be time consuming, to say the least. At that time, my prayer life was not something I found pleasant or rewarding; I felt five minutes was a long time to pray. My thoughts would begin to wander and before I knew it, I was planning the day ahead. For years, I had attended seminars on prayer. I thought some secret formula must exist that would make me a mighty prayer warrior.

The greatest benefit I have received from writing my prayers is the total focus on praying while I am writing. My mind is focused because it is difficult to write and think of other things at the same time. Also, the Holy Spirit directs my praying when my mind is tuned in to God. My faith grows as I go back through my journal and highlight the many answers to prayer in my life.

God has taught me many truths through journaling. I have learned to praise Him in all things. Trials in my life may seem like roadblocks to me, but God sees them as stepping-stones to victory and spiritual growth. Journaling has taught me that God hears and answers all my prayers. When I pray within the framework of God's will, His answer is always a re-sounding yes! When God tells me no, He does so because I have asked something contrary to His will for my life. Many times His no is only "Wait, My child—the timing is not yet right."

Another lesson I learned when writing my prayers is how the Holy Spirit brings to mind sin that hinders my fellowship with God. Sin in me affects everyone I meet. I have learned that by confessing and turning from my sin, I am immediately restored and able to be used in God's service.

Thanksgiving is a very important part of my prayers. While praise is expressing gratitude for who God *is,* thanksgiving is gratitude to God for what He *does.* If we, as earthly parents, love to hear the words "thank you" from our children, how much more God wants us to thank Him for His blessings. God's greatest blessings do not cost a penny. Money can't buy a glorious sunset or a walk on the beach. Good health is a blessing many people would pay much to attain. God blesses us in hundreds of ways each day. I praise God for who He *is* and thank Him for what He *does* in my life.

God has also taught me the importance of intercession in my life as a Christian. The Holy Spirit often breaks loose in others' lives as a discernable result of the prayers of believing Christians. What a joy to see healing and restoration take place in the lives of those we love and know.

Because of what God can do in your life, I recommend that you begin writing your prayers during your participation in First Place 4 Health. The prayer journal is designed to assist you. My prayer is that God will use this process to help you focus your attention on Him as you pray. God bless you as you begin writing your prayers.

—Carole Lewis

prayer journal
sample entry

Use the *First Place 4 Health Prayer Journal* to record your personal prayers and thoughts. You might like to include some of the following: your prayers to God, your praise and thankfulness to God, confessions of sin, and personal requests. Write as much or as little as you like—quality, not quantity, is what matters. Here is a sample prayer journal entry to get you started:

1/25/08

Dear Lord,

I praise You today, for You are my Creator! You are holy, righteous and just. I love You and want to seek You first today in all that I do. You are my all!

Lord, You have my heart, and You know all of my ways. Father, forgive me for being so selfish and not reaching out to those around me. I have been caught up in my own problems and haven't been concerned about those around me. Lord, today I commit to You that I will reach out in love to Martha, my fellow First Place 4 Health group member.

Thank You, Lord, for giving me such caring and loving friends and family. They are a gift from You. Lord, I ask that You would be with me when I reach out to Martha, and I trust that You will provide a way for me to minister to her.

Lord, put a guard over my mouth today and give me eyes to see the way of escape from the temptations I will face today as I eat out with my coworkers. I love You, Lord, and I want to live a life that pleases You. Thank You for sending Jesus to save me from my sins so that I can be in a right relationship with You. I offer this prayer to You in Jesus' name and the power of His Holy Spirit.

Your daughter,

Nancy

what is Scripture?

Scripture—the Bible—is the divinely inspired Word of God. The Bible contains the very thoughts and words of our everlasting, almighty, all-powerful God. Scripture is not simply wise sayings, inspirational stories or the Good Book. Second Timothy 3:16-17 describes the Bible this way:

All Scripture is God-breathed and is useful for teaching, rebuking, correcting and training in righteousness, so that the man of God may be thoroughly equipped for every good work.

The phrase "God-breathed" means "inspired." This means that God is the author of Scripture, although He used humans to write it down. Second Peter 1:21 also talks about this:

For prophecy never had its origin in the will of man, but men spoke from God as they were carried along by the Holy Spirit.

Note that *all* of Scripture is useful. This means that you can read any portion of the Bible, and you will in some way benefit from it. Whether you are seeking wisdom, consolation, encouragement, strength or help, the Bible can be a familiar companion that will speak God's words to you.

The Word of God is alive, because with the Word of God comes the influence of the Holy Spirit. When we talk about the Holy Spirit's ability to apply the pages of Scripture to our lives, we're not talking about magic; we're talking about the fact that God is alive and He uses the very pages of Scripture to speak to us and transform our life and heart when we read and study the Bible:

For the word of God is living and active. Sharper than any double-edged sword, it penetrates even to dividing soul and spirit, joints and marrow; it judges the thoughts and attitudes of the heart (Hebrews 4:12).

As you read the Bible on a consistent and regular basis, your personal relationship with your heavenly Father will become deeper and more meaningful. Prayer is speaking to God, but Scripture reading is God speaking to you.

Although your natural inclination is to get up each day and approach the world on your own, the better way to start each day is to let Scripture focus your view so that you can see the world through the eyes of Christ. Thus, the worldly pressures that likely and inevitably cause a variety of anxieties will be lessened.

Matthew 5:13-14 invites you to be "salt" and "light" in your world—to be someone who makes an impact for truth. Being salt and light means that although you recognize culture's pull, you choose to follow the truth regardless of what culture tells you. Christ's invitation is radical. He wants you to know the truth, be set free by the truth and help others to be set free by the truth. There's only one way to do that. To know what truth is, you need to read God's Word.

When you know Scripture, you can align your desires with truth. Your heart's desires will be for good things, not for things that harm you. When other voices tell you which way you should go, Scripture helps you stand for truth in the midst of those voices. Scripture attacks unhealthy practices and changes you from the inside out so that real change can occur in lasting ways.

READING SCRIPTURE

Begin reading God's Word on a daily basis, and ask God to give you a love for His Word. If you are unfamiliar with the Bible, you might begin by reading the Gospel of John. Read this Gospel several times until you understand what it says; then continue with another book of the Bible. Another good and practical place to start reading is the book of Proverbs.

If you like, you can use a one-year Bible (a variety of these are available at most Christian bookstores) for your systematic reading. In most one-year Bibles, each day's Scripture entry has passages of God's Word selected from the Old Testament, the New Testament and the books of Psalms and Proverbs.

Or you could use the First Place 4 Health Scripture Reading Plan, which lists both Old and New Testament passages to read each day. (You will find the First Place 4 Health plan located on the following pages of this guide.)

As you read, ask God to give you insight from His Word to help you in the activities of your day. Sometimes the Holy Spirit might impress you to stop and reread a particular verse. After you read that verse a few times, God may give you insight into a current problem you're experiencing. He can actually speak to you through a particular verse or passage from His Word.

Remember that there is no right or wrong way to read God's Word. The key is simply to begin.

Scripture reading plan

The following plan will guide you through an Old Testament and New Testament passage each day. You will read through the Bible in one year, if you follow this plan. Each reading will take approximately 15 to 30 minutes to complete each day.

January

1 Genesis 1—3; Matthew 1
2 Genesis 4—6; Matthew 2:1-12
3 Genesis 7—8; Matthew 2:13-23
4 Genesis 9—11; Matthew 3
5 Genesis 12—14; Matthew 4:1-11
6 Genesis 15—17; Matthew 4:12-25
7 Genesis 18—19; Matthew 5:1-16
8 Genesis 20—22; Matthew 5:17-48
9 Genesis 23—24; Matthew 6:1-18
10 Genesis 25—27; Matthew 6:19-34
11 Genesis 28—29; Matthew 7:1-14
12 Genesis 30—31; Matthew 7:15-29
13 Genesis 32—33; Matthew 8:1-17
14 Genesis 34—36; Matthew 8:18-34
15 Genesis 37—38; Matthew 9:1-26
16 Genesis 39—40; Matthew 9:27-38
17 Genesis 41—42; Matthew 10
18 Genesis 43—45; Matthew 11:1-19
19 Genesis 46—47; Matthew 11:20-30
20 Genesis 48—50; Matthew 12:1-21
21 Exodus 1—2; Matthew 12:22-50
22 Exodus 3—4; Matthew 13:1-23
23 Exodus 5—7; Matthew 13:24-58
24 Exodus 8—9; Matthew 14:1-21
25 Exodus 10—11; Matthew 14:22-36
26 Exodus 12—13; Matthew 15:1-20
27 Exodus 14—15; Matthew 15:21-39
28 Exodus 16—18; Matthew 16:1-12
29 Exodus 19—21; Matthew 16:13-28
30 Exodus 22—23; Matthew 17:1-13
31 Exodus 24—26; Matthew 17:14-27

February

1 Exodus 27—28; Matthew 18:1-20
2 Exodus 29—30; Matthew 18:21-35
3 Exodus 31—32; Matthew 19:1-15
4 Exodus 33—34; Matthew 19:16-30
5 Exodus 35—36; Matthew 20:1-16
6 Exodus 37—38; Matthew 20:17-34
7 Exodus 39—40; Matthew 21:1-22
8 Leviticus 1—3; Matthew 21:23-46
9 Leviticus 4—5; Matthew 22:1-14
10 Leviticus 6—8; Matthew 22:15-46
11 Leviticus 9—10; Matthew 23
12 Leviticus 11—13; Matthew 24:1-31
13 Leviticus 14—15; Matthew 24:32-51
14 Leviticus 16—18; Matthew 25:1-30
15 Leviticus 19—20; Matthew 25:31-46
16 Leviticus 21—23; Matthew 26:1-35
17 Leviticus 24—25; Matthew 26:36-56
18 Leviticus 26—27; Matthew 26:57-75
19 Numbers 1—2; Matthew 27:1-31
20 Numbers 3—4; Matthew 27:32-66
21 Numbers 5—6; Matthew 28
22 Numbers 7; Mark 1:1-15
23 Numbers 8—10; Mark 1:16-45
24 Numbers 11—12; Mark 2:1-12
25 Numbers 13—14; Mark 2:13-28
26 Numbers 15—16; Mark 3:1-12
27 Numbers 17—18; Mark 3:13-35
28 Numbers 19—20; Mark 4:1-20
29 Numbers 21; Mark 4:21-41

March

1 Numbers 22—24; Mark 5:1-20
2 Numbers 25—26; Mark 5:21-43
3 Numbers 27—29; Mark 6:1-13
4 Numbers 30—31; Mark 6:14-29
5 Numbers 32—33; Mark 6:30-56
6 Numbers 34—36; Mark 7:1-23
7 Deuteronomy 1—2; Mark 7:24-37
8 Deuteronomy 3—4; Mark 8:1-10
9 Deuteronomy 5—6; Mark 8:11-26
10 Deuteronomy 7—9; Mark 8:27-38
11 Deuteronomy 10—11; Mark 9:1-13
12 Deuteronomy 12—14; Mark 9:14-29
13 Deuteronomy 15—17; Mark 9:30-50
14 Deuteronomy 18—20; Mark 10:1-16
15 Deuteronomy 21—23; Mark 10:17-31
16 Deuteronomy 24—26; Mark 10:32-52
17 Deuteronomy 27—28; Mark 11:1-11
18 Deuteronomy 29—30; Mark 11:12-33
19 Deuteronomy 31—32; Mark 12:1-12
20 Deuteronomy 33—34; Mark 12:13-27
21 Joshua 1—2; Mark 12:28-44
22 Joshua 3—4; Mark 13:1-13
23 Joshua 5—6; Mark 13:14-37
24 Joshua 7—8; Mark 14:1-11
25 Joshua 9—10; Mark 14:12-31

26 Joshua 11—12; Mark 14:32-52
27 Joshua 13—15; Mark 14:53-72
28 Joshua 16—18; Mark 15:1-15
29 Joshua 19—20; Mark 15:16-39
30 Joshua 21—22; Mark 15:40-47
31 Joshua 23—24; Mark 16

April

1 Judges 1—3; Luke 1:1-25
2 Judges 4—5; Luke 1:26-38
3 Judges 6; Luke 1:39-56
4 Judges 7—8; Luke 1:57-80
5 Judges 9; Luke 2:1-20
6 Judges 10—12; Luke 2:21-40
7 Judges 13—15; Luke 2:41-52
8 Judges 16; Luke 3:1-20
9 Judges 17—18; Luke 3:21-38
10 Judges 19—20; Luke 4:1-13
11 Judges 21; Luke 4:14-32
12 Ruth 1—2; Luke 4:33-44
13 Ruth 3—4; Luke 5:1-26
14 1 Samuel 1—2; Luke 5:27-39
15 1 Samuel 3—4; Luke 6:1-11
16 1 Samuel 5—6; Luke 6:12-49
17 1 Samuel 7—8; Luke 7:1-17
18 1 Samuel 9—10; Luke 7:18-35
19 1 Samuel 11—13; Luke 7:36-50
20 1 Samuel 14—15; Luke 8:1-18
21 1 Samuel 16—17; Luke 8:19-39
22 1 Samuel 18—19; Luke 8:40-56
23 1 Samuel 20—21; Luke 9:1-17
24 1 Samuel 22—23; Luke 9:18-45
25 1 Samuel 24—25; Luke 9:46-62
26 1 Samuel 26—27; Luke 10:1-24
27 1 Samuel 28—29; Luke 10:25-42
28 1 Samuel 30—31; Luke 11:1-13
29 2 Samuel 1—2; Luke 11:14-28
30 2 Samuel 3—4; Luke 11:29-54

May

1 2 Samuel 5—6; Luke 12:1-12
2 2 Samuel 7—8; Luke 12:13-34
3 2 Samuel 9—10; Luke 12:35-59
4 2 Samuel 11—12; Luke 13:1-17
5 2 Samuel 13—14; Luke 13:18-35
6 2 Samuel 15—16; Luke 14:1-24
7 2 Samuel 17—18; Luke 14:25-35
8 2 Samuel 19—20; Luke 15
9 2 Samuel 21—22; Luke 16:1-18
10 2 Samuel 23—24; Luke 16:19-31

11 1 Kings 1—2; Luke 17:1-19
12 1 Kings 3—4; Luke 17:20-37
13 1 Kings 5—6; Luke 18:1-17
14 1 Kings 7—8; Luke 18:18-43
15 1 Kings 9—11; Luke 19:1-27
16 1 Kings 12—13; Luke 19:28-48
17 1 Kings 14—15; Luke 20:1-26
18 1 Kings 16—17; Luke 20:27-47
19 1 Kings 18—19; Luke 21:1-28
20 1 Kings 20—21; Luke 21:29-38
21 1 Kings 22; Luke 22:1-23
22 2 Kings 1—3; Luke 22:24-53
23 2 Kings 4—5; Luke 22:54-71
24 2 Kings 6—7; Luke 23:1-25
25 2 Kings 8—9; Luke 23:26-43
26 2 Kings 10—11; Luke 23:44-56
27 2 Kings 12—13; Luke 24:1-12
28 2 Kings 14—15; Luke 24:13-53
29 2 Kings 16—17; John 1:1-18
30 2 Kings 18—20; John 1:19-51
31 2 Kings 21—23; John 2

June

1 2 Kings 24—25; John 3:1-21
2 1 Chronicles 1—2; John 3:22-36
3 1 Chronicles 3—4; John 4:1-42
4 1 Chronicles 5—6; John 4:43-54
5 1 Chronicles 7—8; John 5:1-15
6 1 Chronicles 9—10; John 5:16-47
7 1 Chronicles 11—12; John 6:1-15
8 1 Chronicles 13—15; John 6:16-40
9 1 Chronicles 16—17; John 6:41-71
10 1 Chronicles 18—19; John 7:1-36
11 1 Chronicles 20—21; John 7:37-52
12 1 Chronicles 22—24; John 8:1-11
13 1 Chronicles 25—27; John 8:12-59
14 1 Chronicles 28—29; John 9
15 2 Chronicles 1—2; John 10:1-21
16 2 Chronicles 3—4; John 10:22-42
17 2 Chronicles 5—6; John 11
18 2 Chronicles 7—9; John 12:1-19
19 2 Chronicles 10—12; John 12:20-50
20 2 Chronicles 13—16; John 13
21 2 Chronicles 17—19; John 14
22 2 Chronicles 20—21; John 15
23 2 Chronicles 22—23; John 16
24 2 Chronicles 24—25; John 17
25 2 Chronicles 26—27; John 18
26 2 Chronicles 28—29; John 19:1-16
27 2 Chronicles 30—31; John 19:17-42

28 2 Chronicles 32; John 20:1-18
29 2 Chronicles 33—34; John 20:19-31
30 2 Chronicles 35—36; John 21

July

1 Ezra 1—2; Acts 1
2 Ezra 3—4; Acts 2
3 Ezra 5—6; Acts 3
4 Ezra 7—8; Acts 4:1-22
5 Ezra 9—10; Acts 4:23-37
6 Nehemiah 1—3; Acts 5
7 Nehemiah 4—6; Acts 6
8 Nehemiah 7—9; Acts 7
9 Nehemiah 10—11; Acts 8:1-25
10 Nehemiah 12—13; Acts 8:26-40
11 Esther 1—2; Acts 9:1-22
12 Esther 3—6; Acts 9:23-43
13 Esther 7—10; Acts 10:1-23
14 Job 1—3; Acts 10:24-48
15 Job 4—7; Acts 11
16 Job 8—10; Acts 12
17 Job 11—14; Acts 13:1-12
18 Job 15—17; Acts 13:13-52
19 Job 18—21; Acts 14
20 Job 22—24; Acts 15
21 Job 25—28; Acts 16:1-15
22 Job 29—31; Acts 16:16-40
23 Job 32—34; Acts 17:1-15
24 Job 35—37; Acts 17:16-34
25 Job 38—39; Acts 18
26 Job 40—42; Acts 19:1-20
27 Psalms 1—6; Acts 19:21-41
28 Psalms 7—12; Acts 20:1-16
29 Psalms 13—18; Acts 20:17-38
30 Psalms 19—24; Acts 21:1-16
31 Psalms 25—30; Acts 21:17-40

August

1 Psalms 31—36; Acts 22
2 Psalms 37—41; Acts 23
3 Psalms 42—47; Acts 24
4 Psalms 48—53; Acts 25
5 Psalms 54—58; Acts 26
6 Psalms 59—64; Acts 27
7 Psalms 65—68; Acts 28:1-15
8 Psalms 69—72; Acts 28:16-31
9 Psalms 73—77; Romans 1:1-17
10 Psalms 78—80; Romans 1:18-32
11 Psalms 81—86; Romans 2
12 Psalms 87—89; Romans 3

13   Psalms 90—95; Romans 4
14   Psalms 96—102; Romans 5
15   Psalms 103—106; Romans 6
16   Psalms 107—111; Romans 7
17   Psalms 112—118; Romans 8:1-17
18   Psalms 119:1-88; Romans 8:18-39
19   Psalms 119:89-176; Romans 9
20   Psalms 120—129; Romans 10
21   Psalms 130—136; Romans 11
22   Psalms 137—140; Romans 12
23   Psalms 141—145; Romans 13
24   Psalms 146—150; Romans 14
25   Proverbs 1—3; Romans 15
26   Proverbs 4—6; Romans 16
27   Proverbs 7—9; 1 Corinthians 1
28   Proverbs 10—12; 1 Corinthians 2
29   Proverbs 13—14; 1 Corinthians 3
30   Proverbs 15—17; 1 Corinthians 4
31   Proverbs 18—20; 1 Corinthians 5

September

1   Proverbs 21—23; 1 Corinthians 6
2   Proverbs 24—26; 1 Corinthians 7
3   Proverbs 27—29; 1 Corinthians 8
4   Proverbs 30—31; 1 Corinthians 9
5   Ecclesiastes 1—3; 1 Corinthians 10
6   Ecclesiastes 4—7; 1 Corinthians 11
7   Ecclesiastes 8—12; 1 Corinthians 12
8   Song of Songs 1—4; 1 Corinthians 13
9   Song of Songs 5—8; 1 Corinthians 14
10   Isaiah 1—4; 1 Corinthians 15
11   Isaiah 5—7; 1 Corinthians 16
12   Isaiah 8—9; 2 Corinthians 1
13   Isaiah 10—12; 2 Corinthians 2
14   Isaiah 13—14; 2 Corinthians 3
15   Isaiah 15—18; 2 Corinthians 4
16   Isaiah 19—22; 2 Corinthians 5
17   Isaiah 23—25; 2 Corinthians 6
18   Isaiah 26—29; 2 Corinthians 7
19   Isaiah 30—32; 2 Corinthians 8
20   Isaiah 33—35; 2 Corinthians 9
21   Isaiah 36—39; 2 Corinthians 10
22   Isaiah 40—41; 2 Corinthians 11
23   Isaiah 42—43; 2 Corinthians 12
24   Isaiah 44—47; 2 Corinthians 13
25   Isaiah 48—50; Galatians 1
26   Isaiah 51—53; Galatians 2
27   Isaiah 54—57; Galatians 3
28   Isaiah 58—60; Galatians 4
29   Isaiah 61—63; Galatians 5
30   Isaiah 64—66; Galatians 6

October

1   Jeremiah 1; Ephesians 1
2   Jeremiah 2; Ephesians 2
3   Jeremiah 3—4; Ephesians 3
4   Jeremiah 5—6; Ephesians 4
5   Jeremiah 7—8; Ephesians 5
6   Jeremiah 9—10; Ephesians 6
7   Jeremiah 11—12; Philippians 1
8   Jeremiah 13—14; Philippians 2
9   Jeremiah 15—17; Philippians 3
10   Jeremiah 18—19; Philippians 4
11   Jeremiah 20—21; Colossians 1
12   Jeremiah 22—23; Colossians 2
13   Jeremiah 24—25; Colossians 3
14   Jeremiah 26; Colossians 4
15   Jeremiah 27—28; 1 Thessalonians 1
16   Jeremiah 29—30; 1 Thessalonians 2
17   Jeremiah 31; 1 Thessalonians 3
18   Jeremiah 32; 1 Thessalonians 4
19   Jeremiah 33—34; 1 Thessalonians 5
20   Jeremiah 35—36; 2 Thessalonians 1
21   Jeremiah 37—38; 2 Thessalonians 2
22   Jeremiah 39—41; 2 Thessalonians 3
23   Jeremiah 42—43; 1 Timothy 1
24   Jeremiah 44—45; 1 Timothy 2
25   Jeremiah 46—47; 1 Timothy 3
26   Jeremiah 48; 1 Timothy 4
27   Jeremiah 49; 1 Timothy 5
28   Jeremiah 50; 1 Timothy 6
29   Jeremiah 51; 2 Timothy 1
30   Jeremiah 52; 2 Timothy 2
31   Lamentations 1; 2 Timothy 3

November

1   Lamentations 2; 2 Timothy 4
2   Lamentations 3; Titus 1
3   Lamentations 4; Titus 2
4   Lamentations 5; Titus 3
5   Ezekiel 1—2; Philemon
6   Ezekiel 3—5; Hebrews 1
7   Ezekiel 6—7; Hebrews 2
8   Ezekiel 8—10; Hebrews 3
9   Ezekiel 11—12; Hebrews 4
10   Ezekiel 13—14; Hebrews 5
11   Ezekiel 15—16; Hebrews 6
12   Ezekiel 17—18; Hebrews 7
13   Ezekiel 19—20; Hebrews 8
14   Ezekiel 21—22; Hebrews 9
15   Ezekiel 23—24; Hebrews 10
16   Ezekiel 25—26; Hebrews 11
17   Ezekiel 27—28; Hebrews 12
18   Ezekiel 29—30; Hebrews 13
19   Ezekiel 31—32; James 1
20   Ezekiel 33—34; James 2
21   Ezekiel 35—37; James 3
22   Ezekiel 38—39; James 4
23   Ezekiel 40—41; James 5
24   Ezekiel 42—43; 1 Peter 1
25   Ezekiel 44—46; 1 Peter 2
26   Ezekiel 47—48; 1 Peter 3
27   Daniel 1; 1 Peter 4
28   Daniel 2; 1 Peter 5
29   Daniel 3; 2 Peter 1
30   Daniel 4; 2 Peter 2

December

1   Daniel 5—6; 2 Peter 3
2   Daniel 7—8; 1 John 1
3   Daniel 9; 1 John 2
4   Daniel 10—12; 1 John 3
5   Hosea 1—3; 1 John 4
6   Hosea 4—6; 1 John 5
7   Hosea 7—8; 2 John
8   Hosea 9—10; 3 John
9   Hosea 11—12; Jude
10   Hosea 13—14; Revelation 1
11   Joel; Revelation 2
12   Amos 1—2; Revelation 3
13   Amos 3—4; Revelation 4
14   Amos 5—7; Revelation 5
15   Amos 8—9; Revelation 6
16   Obadiah; Revelation 7
17   Jonah; Revelation 8
18   Micah 1—2; Revelation 9
19   Micah 3—4; Revelation 10
20   Micah 5—7; Revelation 11
21   Nahum; Revelation 12
22   Habakkuk; Revelation 13
23   Zephaniah; Revelation 14
24   Haggai; Revelation 15
25   Zechariah 1—3; Revelation 16
26   Zechariah 4—5; Revelation 17
27   Zechariah 6—8; Revelation 18
28   Zechariah 9—11; Revelation 19
29   Zechariah 12—14; Revelation 20
30   Malachi 1—2; Revelation 21
31   Malachi 3—4; Revelation 22

studying
Scripture

Bible study is closely linked with reading Scripture every day. What distinguishes each First Place 4 Health Bible study is that in addition to reading the Bible, you study a specific area of the Bible for an entire week and use discussion questions to help you learn what the text means. Each First Place 4 Health Bible study book contains 10 weeks of lessons. Each week has five days of questions related to the Scriptures you are studying and then two days reserved for reflection on what you have learned that week and how you have applied what you have learned.

When you study the Bible—when you open it up and mine the depths of its contents—you will find a depth of living you won't find by doing anything else. This depth is crucial for the balance that's so necessary in your life. When you truly know who the Lord is—when you diligently dig in to what the Lord says about Himself and the plan He has for you as found in the pages of Scripture—you will fall in love with the God of wonders. Christ will become like a good friend with whom you have real communion, and the rest of your life will naturally and spiritually fall into place.

What does studying the Bible possibly have to do with losing weight? Much more than you might think. Weight loss is not just a physical issue; it's also a spiritual issue. True change starts in your spirit, your mind, your emotions and your *body* when you begin to ingest truth into your life; and God is the ultimate source of all truth.

Know the Truth

When you open your Bible and study it, you have the opportunity to know what Bible passages really mean. You can see for yourself what Scripture says in the context in which it was written. "Context" takes into account the specific background and circumstances of a passage. It gives you a correct framework for knowing what a particular passage is talking about.

For instance, some portions of Scripture were addressed to a specific group of people during a specific time in history. Other portions were written as poetry. Some passages use metaphors or similes; for example, when Psalm 57:1 describes how we can "take refuge in the shadow of [God's] *wings,*" the writer is not suggesting that God is an actual bird; rather, this is an image of God's protection.

Know Christ

It's far easier to call yourself a Christian than it is to follow Christ. To truly know His words and what He's like, you need to spend time with Him. To know the depth and substance of what you truly say you believe means that you have to sit down and explore who Jesus Christ is and the path He invites you to walk.

Think of studying Scripture as having a personal conversation with God. It's not casual conversation; it's serious business.

Get Balanced

The First Place 4 Health topical Bible studies directly relate to your life, because the studies are targeted to areas in which we all struggle. Using one of the First Place 4 Health Bible studies to explore the Bible on your own throughout the week—and with your First Place 4 Health group once a week—helps you understand the Word of God so that you can apply it to your life.

For example, your group might have a study on resisting temptation, and in that study you will look closely at the words of 1 Corinthians 10:13:

> No temptation has seized you except what is common to man. And God is faithful; he will not let you be tempted beyond what you can bear. But when you are tempted, he will also provide a way out so that you can stand up under it.

What will this verse look like in your life? How will it apply to weight loss? What will it look like in your life the next time you're feeling down and you head to the refrigerator to pick yourself back up? Those are the types of questions you'll discuss with your group in a First Place 4 Health Bible study. There are many First Place 4 Health Bible studies, each written to address a specific topic that is relevant to this life-transforming program. To get the full benefit of First Place 4 Health, study God's Word and then apply the truth of Scripture to your life.

THE COMPONENTS OF BIBLE STUDY

Bible study breaks down into three separate components: observation, interpretation and application.

Observation

Observation simply means looking at the text. When you sit down to study Scripture, first read through the passage several times. Don't jump to conclusions right away. Ask these questions: Who's talking? Who's listening? Where is this taking place? What's going on? When did this happen?

Interpretation

Interpretation means correctly determining what a passage means. There are a variety of criteria for determining this, but here are three good rules of thumb:

1. **Interpret a passage in light of its style.** For example, there are many Bible passages written as songs or poems; when you read these, note any play on words, the use of any particular images and the use of any figures of speech (similes, metaphors, and so on). You will read other Bible passages that were written as history (for example, the book of Acts); when you read these, keep in mind that these events happened in a specific place and time.

2. **Interpret a passage in its specific context.** Read at least the five verses before and the five verses after the passage you're seeking to interpret. What does the passage you want to interpret mean within the flow of the chapter and/or the book as a whole?

3. **Interpret a passage in light of the rest of Scripture.** Compare the passage with the same or similar verses in other books of the Bible. There is a marvelous harmony within the Bible.

Application

Application means putting to use in your life what you've learned from the observation and interpretation components. Is there a promise to believe? An example to follow? A sin to avoid? Ask yourself, *How will my life be different if I apply what this Scripture passage says?*

BIBLE STUDY TOOLS

You may also want to use some additional resources outside of the First Place 4 Health studies. There are many resources available that will enhance your study time in God's Word, including different Bible translations and other study tools. You may want to acquire these various resources over a period of time.

Different Bible Translations

Choose a Bible translation that you enjoy reading and using. The First Place 4 Health Bible studies use the *New International Version,* but there are also many other excellent modern translations, such as the *English Standard Version*, the *New Century Version*, the *New Living Translation* and the *New American Standard. THE MESSAGE*, a translation of the Bible by Eugene Peterson, is a creative and moving modern paraphrase; it was translated concept by concept rather than word by word from the original languages. Although reading a paraphrase translation such as *THE MESSAGE* or the *Living Bible* is enjoyable, do your study from one of the word-by-word translations.

A Parallel Bible

A parallel Bible includes two to four translations right next to each other in columns. When you study God's Word, it is often useful to read several different translations, because each one gives a different insight into each verse.

A Concordance

A concordance is a book that contains an alphabetized list of all the words found in the Bible. If you can just remember a part of a verse but you don't know where it's found, you can look up in a concordance just one main word from that verse and find the verse. A concordance will also help you study different topics or words from the Bible.

A Bible Commentary

Bible commentaries are written by scholars to explain passages and to provide a broader understanding of Bible passages. There are a wide variety of commentaries available, either in a single volume for the entire Bible or in multiple volumes for each book of the Bible.

One good commentary is *The Bible Knowledge Commentary: An Exposition of the Scriptures by Dallas Seminary Faculty* by John F. Walvoord and Roy B. Zuck, two scholars from Dallas Theological Seminary. This excellent two-volume set will help you understand the meaning of the text without any complicated jargon.

A Bible Dictionary

A Bible dictionary will give you insight into the cultural background of the Bible and help you understand definitions of difficult terms like "atonement" and "sanctification."

A Study Bible

As an alternative to several of these resources, consider buying a good study Bible. Like the variety of Bible translations, there are many different study Bibles available. Visit your local Christian bookstore, and look through the various types of study Bibles. Talk with a salesperson to make an informed decision. (The *NIV Life Application Study Bible* is a very good and practical resource.)

Bible Study Websites

Almost anything in print today can also be found in an electronic version, either through a publisher or online. One excellent resource is e-Sword (www.e-sword.net), which offers a variety of Bible versions, commentaries, dictionaries and study notes—all for free.

Another good website is provided by the International Bible Society at www.ibs.org. This site offers online Bibles and search tools, as well as summaries and study helps.

Bible Gateway offers different Bible versions, Bible concordances, study helps and search tools for free. Find them at www.bibles.net.

sharing
your faith!

Nothing is more effective in drawing someone to Jesus than sharing personal life experiences. People are more open to the good news of Jesus Christ when they see faith in action. Personal faith stories are simple and effective ways to share what Christ is doing in your life, because they show firsthand how Christ makes a difference. Sharing your faith story has an added benefit: It builds you up in your faith, too!

Is your experience in First Place 4 Health providing you opportunities to share with others what God is doing in your life? If you answered yes, then you have a personal faith story! If you do not have a personal faith story, perhaps it is because you don't know Jesus Christ as your personal Lord and Savior. Read through "Steps to Becoming a Christian" (which is the next chapter) and begin today to give Christ first place in your life.

Creativity and preparation in using opportunities to share a word or story about Jesus is an important part of the Christian life. Is Jesus helping you in a special way? Are you achieving a level of success or peace that you haven't experienced in other attempts to lose weight, exercise regularly or eat healthier? As people see you making changes and achieving success, they may ask you how you are doing it. How will—or do—you respond?

Remember, your story is unique and it may allow others to see what Christ is doing in your life. It may also help to bring Christ into the life of another person.

PERSONAL STATEMENTS OF FAITH

First Place 4 Health gives you a great opportunity to communicate your faith and express what God is doing in your life. Be ready to use your own personal statement of faith whenever the opportunity presents itself. Personal statements of faith should be short and fit naturally into a conversation. They don't require or expect any action or response from the listener. The goal is not to get another person to change but simply to help you communicate who you are and what's important to you. Here are some examples of short statements of faith that you might use when someone asks what you are doing to lose weight:

- "I've been meeting with a group at my church. We pray together, support each other, learn about nutrition and study the Bible."
- "It's amazing how Bible study and prayer are helping me lose weight and eat healthier."
- "I've had a lot of support from a group I meet with at church."
- "I'm relying more on God to help me make changes in my lifestyle."

Begin keeping a list of your meaningful experiences as you go through the First Place 4 Health program. Also notice what is happening in the lives of others. Use the following questions to help you prepare short personal statements and stories of faith:

1 What is God doing in your life physically, mentally, emotionally and spiritually?

2 How has your relationship with God changed? Is it more intimate or personal?

3 How is prayer, Bible study and/or the support of others helping you achieve your goals for a healthy weight and good nutrition?

WRITING YOUR PERSONAL FAITH STORY

Write a brief story about how God is working in your life through First Place 4 Health. Use your story to help you share with others what's happening in your life. Use the following questions to help develop your story:

1. Why did you join First Place 4 Health? What specific circumstances led you to a Christ-centered health and weight-loss program? What were you feeling when you joined?

2. What was your relationship with Christ when you started First Place 4 Health? What is it now?

3. Has your experience in First Place 4 Health changed your relationship with Christ? With yourself? With others?

4. How has your relationship with Christ, prayer, Bible study and group support made a difference in your life?

5. What specific verse or passage of Scripture has made a difference in the way you view yourself or your relationship with Christ?

6. What experiences have impacted your life since starting First Place 4 Health?

7. In what ways is Christ working in your life today? In what ways is He meeting your needs?

8. How has Christ worked in other members of your First Place 4 Health group?

Answer the above questions in a few sentences, and then use your answers to help you write your own short personal faith story.

steps to becoming a Christian

Spiritual transformation begins the moment you accept Jesus Christ as your Lord and Savior. Conversely, if you have not been made right with God through the saving sacrifice of Jesus Christ, no amount of study can bring spiritual renewal. "If the Son sets you free you will be free indeed" (John 8:36). Accepting Christ as your Lord and Savior is the essential first step in putting Him first in all things! Without the freedom that comes when you accept Jesus Christ as your personal Lord and Savior, First Place 4 Health will be just another diet and exercise program.

What the Bible Says
- We were made for God.
- God seeks a relationship with each of us.
- God yearns for us to spend eternity with Him in heaven.

The Bad News
Sin separates us from God and eliminates our hope for heaven. (Sin is defined as missing what God wants for our lives. Think of a bull's-eye and the arrows that have missed the center mark; sin means missing God's mark for us.)

The Good News
- Jesus, God's only Son, came to Earth as a human.
- Jesus willingly became our sacrifice by dying on the cross for our sins.
- We cannot save ourselves. Jesus' blood covers all our sins and reconciles us to God.

The Decision
Have you ever made the decision to ask Jesus Christ to be your Savior?

❏ Yes   ❏ No

If you answered yes, use the lines below the following steps to write about your personal experience. If your answer is no, please open your heart to God now. These are five simple steps to take:

1. **Acknowledge that you are a sinner.** "For all have sinned and fall short of the glory of God" (Romans 3:23).

2. **Acknowledge that sin separates you from God.** "For the wages of sin is death, but the gift of God is eternal life in Christ Jesus our Lord" (Romans 6:23).

3. **Acknowledge that Christ died for you.** "But God demonstrates his own love for us in this: While we were still sinners, Christ died for us" (Romans 5:8).

4. **Receive Christ as your Savior.** "If you confess with your mouth 'Jesus is Lord,' and believe in your heart that God raised him from the dead, you will be saved. For it is with your heart that you believe and are justified, and it is with your mouth that you confess and are saved" (Romans 10:9-10).

5. **Now pray these words:** "Dear God, I know I am a sinner and separated from You. I believe You love me and that You sent Jesus to die on the cross for me. I accept You as my Savior and my Lord. Please forgive me of my sin and teach me how to give You first place in my life. Amen."

Mind

LEARN IT

- ◆ Renew your mind. (Scripture memory changes your thoughts so that they align with God's thoughts.)
- ◆ Change your thinking to change how you live. (Weight loss begins in the mind.)
- ◆ Examine your faulty thoughts about food and exercise.
- ◆ Learn to challenge faulty assumptions about your appearance.
- ◆ Replace worry, anxiety and fear with trust in God's love and abundant provision for all your needs.
- ◆ Realize that God has given you everything you need, including enough time.
- ◆ Recognize that temptation is part of being human.
- ◆ Identify your strongholds.

LIVE IT

- ◆ Memorize God's Word by using the First Place 4 Health Scripture memory CDs or by learning Scripture with a friend.
- ◆ Stop negative self-talk and develop a new way of thinking.
- ◆ Embrace healthy eating as a lifestyle.
- ◆ Celebrate the fact that you are fearfully and wonderfully made by God.
- ◆ Use the First Place 4 Health plan for winning over worry.
- ◆ Find time for a healthy you.
- ◆ Resist temptation God's way.
- ◆ Enjoy the freedom Christ died to give you.

God's Word
for your life!

I have hidden your word in my heart that I might not sin against you.

PSALM 119:11

A s you begin to make decisions based on what God's Word teaches you, you'll want to memorize what He has promised to those who trust and follow Him. Second Peter 1:3 tells us that God "has given us everything we need for life and godliness through *our knowledge of Him*" (emphasis added). The Bible provides instruction and encouragement for any area of life in which you may be struggling. If you are dealing with a particular emotion or traumatic life event—fear, discouragement, stress, financial upset, the death of a loved one, a relationship difficulty—you can search through a Bible concordance for Scripture passages that deal with that particular situation. Scripture provides great comfort to those who memorize it.

One of the promises of knowing and obeying God's Word is that it gives you wisdom, insight and understanding above all worldly knowledge (see Psalm 119:97-104). Verses 129-130 of Psalm 119 say, "Your statutes are wonderful; therefore I obey them. The unfolding of your words gives light; it gives understanding to the simple." Now that's a precious promise about guidance for life!

THE VALUE OF SCRIPTURE MEMORY

Scripture memory is an important part of the Christian life, and there are four reasons to memorize Scripture:

1. **To handle difficult situations.** A heartfelt knowledge of God's Word equips us to handle any situation that we might face. Declaring such truth as, "I can do everything through Christ" (see Philippians

46

4:13) and "He will never leave me or forsake me" (see Hebrews 13:5) will enable us to walk through situations with peace and courage.

2. **To overcome temptation.** Luke 4:1-13 describes how Jesus used Scripture to overcome His temptations in the desert (see also Matthew 4:1-11). Knowledge of Scripture and the strength that comes with the ability to use it are important parts of putting on the full armor of God in preparation for spiritual warfare (see Ephesians 6:10-18).

3. **To get guidance.** Psalm 119:105 states that the Word of God "is a lamp to my feet and a light for my path." We learn to hide God's Word in our heart so that His light can direct our decisions and actions throughout our day.

4. **To transform our mind.** "Do not conform any longer to the pattern of this world, but be transformed by the renewing of your mind" (Romans 12:2). Scripture memory allows us to replace a lie with the truth of God's Word.

When Scripture becomes firmly settled in your memory, not only will your thoughts connect with God's thoughts, but you will also be able to honor God with small, everyday decisions as well as big life-impacting ones. Scripture memorization is the key to making a permanent lifestyle change in your thought patterns, which will also bring balance to every other area of your life.

SCRIPTURE MEMORY TIPS

1 Write the verse down, saying it aloud as you write it.

2 Read verses before and after the memory verse for the verse's context.

3 Read the verse several times, emphasizing a different word each time.

4 Connect the Scripture reference to the first few words.

5 Locate patterns, phrases or keywords.

6 Apply the Scripture to circumstances you are now experiencing.

7 Pray the verse, making it personal to your life and inserting your name as the recipient of the promise or teaching. Try that with 1 Corinthians 10:13, inserting "me" and "I" for "you."

8 Review the verse every day until it becomes second nature to think those words whenever your circumstances match its message. The Holy Spirit will bring the verse to mind when you need it most if you will plant it in your memory.

9 Use the First Place 4 Health memory aids, such as the memory verse cards found at the back of each Bible study, and the Scripture Memory CD found in a pocket on the inside back cover of each Bible study. (By using the CDs, you can exercise to music at the same time you are hiding God's Word in your heart.)

SCRIPTURE MEMORIZATION MADE EASY!

What is your learning style? Do you learn by hearing, by sight or by doing? If you learn by hearing—if you are an auditory learner—then singing the Scripture memory verses, reading them aloud or recording them and listening to your recording will be very helpful in the memorization process.

If you are a visual learner, then writing the verses and repeatedly reading through them will cement them in your mind.

If you learn by doing—if you are a tactile learner—then creating motions for the words or using sign language will enable you to more easily recall the verse.

After determining your learning style, link your Scripture memory with a daily task, such as driving to work, walking on a treadmill or eating lunch. Use these daily tasks as opportunities to memorize and review your verses.

Meals at home or out with friends can be used as a time to share the verse you are memorizing with those at your table. You could close your personal email messages by typing in your weekly memory verse; or why not say your memory verse every time you brush your teeth or put on your shoes?

The purpose of Scripture memorization is to be able to apply God's words to your life. If you memorize Scripture using methods that connect with your particular learning style, you will find it easier to hide God's Word in your heart.

a new way
of thinking!

D id you know that you are unable to think a positive thought and a negative thought at the same time? How you think is central to the way you view yourself. Becoming a new creation in Christ means transforming a depraved mind into one that is controlled by the Holy Spirit. Paul referred to this in Romans 8:6: "The mind of sinful man is death, but the mind controlled by the Spirit is life and peace." You can choose either to let the world and its philosophies rule your thoughts or let God rule them. The Bible provides a way to transform your way of thinking.

STEP 1: REARRANGE YOUR THINKING

Words like "always" and "never" can be indicators of what psychologists call imperative thinking—a way of thinking that sets you up for failure. Perhaps a better name would be "stinking thinking." Read the thoughts below. Have you ever found yourself thinking any of the following statements?

- It's no use; I'm a failure.
- Why should I even try again? I know I will never be able to finish _____.
- There may be hope for others, but not for me.
- My boss is right—I'm just lazy.
- See? I blew it again. I'm such a loser.

You can challenge stinking thinking by focusing your thoughts on better things. Philippians 4:8 tells us, "Whatever is true, whatever is noble, whatever is right, whatever is pure, whatever is lovely, whatever is admirable—if anything is excellent or praiseworthy—think about such things."

There is a difference between positive thinking and positive faith. Ephesians 3:20 tells us that God is able to do much more than we can imagine. We can't change by our good intentions alone; we are only truly transformed when we trust in the power of God within us—when we trust His Holy Spirit—and then take steps to walk in God's freedom.

STEP 2: GET RID OF FAULTY ASSUMPTIONS

The following statements are commonly held assumptions. Place a check mark by ones that apply to your thinking.

- ❐ Everything I do should please others.
- ❐ If people around me are unhappy, it's probably my fault.
- ❐ God expects me to finish everything well without making any mistakes.
- ❐ I should not need others' help to succeed.
- ❐ What has happened to me in the past has determined my path for life, and there's nothing I can do about it.
- ❐ If people could see the real me, they probably wouldn't like me.

The more thoughts you checked above, the more you will be hindered in your growth as a new creation in Christ. But it *is* possible to replace those ungodly assumptions with godly truth so that you can continue to grow in Christ.

STEP 3: REPLACE LIES WITH TRUTH

Look at the following chart. In the left-hand column are common lies people believe. In the right-hand column are truths that replace those lies.

LIES	TRUTHS
It's too hard for me to commit to anything. I'm too busy and I don't have time.	*If I commit my way to the Lord and trust in Him, He will give me the time. God is committed to those who are committed to Him (see Proverbs 16:3).*
I'm not good at making wise decisions.	*If I trust in the Lord with all my heart and acknowledge Him in all my ways, He will give me the direction and wisdom that I need (see Proverbs 3:5-6).*
I can't understand God.	*I have been given the mind of Christ (see 1 Corinthians 2:16). I can better understand God with the help of the Holy Spirit and the Bible.*

What lies that need to be replaced with God's truth have you been telling yourself? Ask God to transform your thinking as you begin reading and studying His Word and relying on the Holy Spirit's help (see John 14:26; 16:13).

PRAYER JOURNAL ENTRY

Set up a section in your prayer journal to record, over a period of time, how the Holy Spirit is directing your thinking (see Romans 8:5-6). Use the guidance of the following entries below (greatest challenge this week; lie believed; truth learned) to record how your pattern of thinking is changing as you immerse yourself in God's Word and walk in His truth. (You may want to set up similar sections in your journal for the other areas of your life— body, emotions and spirit—and record, over a period of time, your greatest challenges, lies believed and truths learned in those areas as well.) To begin thinking in this vein, try to recall some recent examples of how you were able to overcome negative self-talk.

My greatest challenge this week in the mental realm (attitudes? relationships?) was _____

_____

_____

_____

The lie(s) I believed (negative self-talk? distractions? lack of understanding?) was _____

_____

_____

_____

The truth I learned that overcame the lie (through meditation on God's Word, through prayer, from Bible study) is _____

_____

_____

_____

Today and in the coming week, I will work on (list an attitude or action connected with a person, place or activity) _____

_____

_____

_____

_____

a new way of
thinking about food

EMBRACE HEALTHY EATING AS A LIFESTYLE

Play the new tape! Think of your healthy food choices as a lifestyle, not as a temporary stop until you can go back to high-fat, high-sugar choices.

Old self-talk tape: *As soon as I get to my goal weight, the first thing I'm going to reward myself with is a big juicy cheeseburger, and I'll top it off with a hot-fudge sundae.*

New self-talk tape: *As soon as I get to my goal weight, I will continue to make healthy food choices. I can have an occasional dessert, but food is no longer a reward. Unhealthy food choices no longer rule me. I am able to enjoy all foods—even an occasional favorite food in moderation—without returning to my old ways of using food to fill the places that have nothing to do with hunger.*

STOP USING FOOD AS A DISTRACTION

Play the new tape! Do you eat by default whenever you're faced with a task you don't want to do? Practice doing part of the task for 10 to 15 minutes, and then see if you still feel the urge to go to the refrigerator.

Old self-talk tape: *Right now I just can't face* _____ [clean the house, pay the bills, create the Excel spreadsheet report due tomorrow—fill in the blank with whatever your dreaded task is]. *I think I'll go get something to eat.*

New self-talk tape: *I'm going to* _____ [clean one bedroom, pay a few bills, do the first section of the report—fill in the blank with your dreaded task] *and see if I'm still hungry after I do that.*

DISCONNECT THE THOUGHT OF FOOD AS A REWARD

Play the new tape! Come up with several nonfood ways to reward your efforts, and enjoy one of those rewards today.

Old self-talk tape: *I've been exercising hard today; I need to eat.*

New self-talk tape: *That exercise was good for my body; now I think I'll relax with a good book.*

YOUR PERSONAL TAPE-OVER

What frequent tape plays in your mind when it comes to your relationship with food? Fill in the first section below with your old mental conversation. Then come up with a new way of talking to yourself, and write it in the second section. In the third section, record a specific action to practice your new self-talk.

Old self-talk tape: _____
_____
_____

New self-talk tape: _____
_____
_____

Play the new tape: _____
_____
_____

THOUGHTS FOR THE JOURNEY

- Before putting food in your mouth, first ask yourself if you're really hungry or if something else is going on in your emotions or thoughts that is causing you to run to food for comfort.

- You can enjoy all foods in moderation, so tape over your diet mentality of deprivation, and replace it with a desire to seek quality and limit quantity.

- If you do blow it, don't beat yourself up; just make the right choices for your next meal or snack.

- Life is a process, and so is your health journey. Approach each day with the attitude that you will do the next right thing—you will make a series of small positive choices every day that will ultimately result in the changes that you desire in body, mind, emotions and spirit.

a healthy
self-image!

Do you not know that your body is a temple of the Holy Spirit,
who is in you, whom you have received from God?

1 CORINTHIANS 6:19

A healthy self-image is an important part of being a new creation in Christ. When you begin to understand what Christ has done for you, your self-talk will begin to change. Let's explore three steps that will help you realize who you truly are in Christ.

STEP 1: REALIZE AND APPRECIATE YOUR UNIQUENESS

It's a proven fact: There is no one else exactly like you! You are uniquely created to be one of a kind. Nothing about you is a mistake. Read the psalmist's words regarding God's creation of your individuality:

> For you created my inmost being; you knit me together in my mother's womb. I praise you because I am fearfully and wonderfully made; your works are wonderful, I know that full well. My frame was not hidden from you when I was made in the secret place. When I was woven together in the depths of the earth, your eyes saw my unformed body. All the days ordained for me were written in your book before one of them came to be (Psalm 139:13-16).

Identify something unique about yourself that sets you apart from others and that you could offer to God for His service. Spend a few moments in prayer, thanking God for your unique design and for His intimate involvement in creating you.

STEP 2: THINK ABOUT WHAT IS TRUE

Another area in which people have many faulty assumptions is their appearance. Take a look at the following faulty assumptions and truths to ponder.

Faulty assumption: *Looks are central to who I am.*

Truth to ponder: *Consider the lives of people such as Corrie ten Boom, Billy Graham and Mother Teresa. Their looks are not the first thing you think of when you admire them.*

Faulty assumption: *The first thing people notice about my appearance are my imperfections.*

Truth to ponder: *Most people notice your best feature first. Remember, we're harder on ourselves than other people are!*

Faulty assumption: *Appearance always reflects the inner person.*

Truth to ponder: *Consider Christ. Scripture tells us there was nothing lovely about His appearance that would draw us to Him* (see Isaiah 53:2).

The next two truths to ponder have been left blank for you to complete.

Faulty assumption: *My appearance is responsible for much of what has happened to me.*

Truth to ponder: _____

_____

_____

Faulty assumption: *The only way I can ever be happy is to change the way I look.*

Truth to ponder: _____

_____

_____

STEP 3: SEE YOUR BODY AS A GIFT

Do a little experiment. Close your eyes and picture yourself. Now suppose you were given the opportunity to ask God to change one thing about your body—what would you ask Him to change?

Now identify at least one thing about your physical body that you really like—not your personality or something inside you, but about your body. That wasn't as easy, was it?

Ask God to begin changing your thoughts about your body. Ask Him to instill in you a sense of wonder for how intricately complex and amazing He has created your body to interact with your brain. You are fearfully and wonderfully made!

winning over worry!

D o you worry about the future—the "what ifs" of life? Are daily responsibilities wearing you down? If you answered yes to either question, worry is adding to your stress level and taking a toll on your health, happiness and effectiveness. Worry can rob us physically, mentally, emotionally and spiritually—but it doesn't have to be that way. God's Word says, "Who of you by worrying can add a single hour to his life?" (Matthew 6:27). "Cast all your anxiety on him because he cares for you" (1 Peter 5:7).

The strain of worry can result in the following negative effects:

- Drawing your focus away from God
- Interference with your relationships
- Feelings of fatigue
- Suppression of the immune system
- Headaches, digestive problems, sleeplessness and depression
- Encouragement of unhealthy habits such as poor nutrition and physical inactivity

A SCRIPTURAL PROMISE

Many times our worries are very real: pressures at work, too much responsibility at home or perhaps financial difficulties. Other times, worry only exists in our mind and our imagination. As the saying goes, 99 percent of what we worry about never happens. What causes you to feel stressed or worried? Are you doing all that you can to eliminate or respond positively to the worries in your life? Are you trusting God to deliver you from your worries? God never promises that you will not experience difficult times, but He does offer a way out:

Come to me, all you who are weary and burdened, and I will give you rest. Take my yoke upon you and learn from me, for I am gentle and humble in heart, and you will find rest for your souls. For my yoke is easy and my burden is light (Matthew 11:28-30).

A PLAN FOR WINNING OVER WORRY

God's prescription for overcoming worry is found in His Word—the Bible.

1. Take Life One Day at a Time

"Therefore do not worry about tomorrow, for tomorrow will worry about itself. Each day has enough trouble of its own" (Matthew 6:34).

Are you managing your time well? Are your goals in line with God's purposes for your life? Are you making time in your life for the important things? In Matthew 6:34, Jesus doesn't tell us not to *think about* tomorrow; He tells us not to *worry about* tomorrow! Planning and preparation will help eliminate some stress. Keeping a calendar or schedule will help you organize your time. Learn to say no more often, and eliminate those things that are less important. Keep the big picture of your life in front of you.

2. Take Time to Rest and Relax

"Come with me by yourselves to a quiet place and get some rest" (Mark 6:31).

Take at least 15 to 20 minutes every day to do something relaxing. Choose what works best for you: sit quietly, breathe deeply, take a walk, read, meditate on Scripture or pray. Imagine a soothing scene in your mind while listening to peaceful music; progressive relaxation involves tightening and relaxing each muscle group in your body as you lie comfortably and breathe deeply.

3. Take Care of Yourself

"Do you not know that your body is a temple of the Holy Spirit, who is in you, whom you have received from God? You are not your own; you were bought at a price. Therefore honor God with your body" (1 Corinthians 6:19-20).

Are you making time for regular physical activity? Are you following a healthy eating plan and getting adequate sleep? Do your poor health habits or feelings about your body contribute to the worry in your life? Physical activity is a great way to relieve worry. A physically fit body responds better to the stresses of life. Regular endurance exercises may even trigger the relaxation response by releasing feel-good hormones called endorphins. Do what you enjoy—walk, swim, ride a bike or jog. Any activity that gets your muscles moving and increases your heart rate can be helpful.

4. Build Supportive Relationships

"A friend loves at all times and a brother is born for adversity" (Proverbs 17:17).

Do you have a close network of family and friends who can help you in times of stress? Getting wise counsel can make you feel better and help you put things in perspective. Make sure you establish supportive relationships with positive people. Sharing your burdens and concerns with others is biblical (see Galatians 6:2). We need each other in good times and bad.

THE MIND-BODY CONNECTION

Whenever you're feeling stressed, personalize the following verses by inserting your name where shown:

> [Your name], do not be anxious about anything, but in everything, by prayer and petition, with thanksgiving, present your requests to God. And the peace of God, which transcends all understanding, will guard your [heart] and [mind] in Christ Jesus (Philippians 4:6-7).

> [Your name], peace I leave with you; my peace I give you. I do not give to you as the world gives. [Your name], do not let your [heart] be troubled and do not be afraid (John 14:27).

As you meditate on these verses and breathe deeply, think about the words "peace," "do not be anxious" and "do not let your [heart] be troubled." Try to fill your lungs from the top to the bottom, and as you breathe out, feel your muscles relax. What you're experiencing is the body's relaxation response—God's design to help the body overcome the effects of worry, stress and anxiety.

what is it time for?

Too much to do and not enough time? Wondering how you will ever find time to work the First Place 4 Health program into your already jam-packed schedule? When we first begin to incorporate the various components of the First Place 4 Health lifestyle into an already over-committed time schedule, we quickly find there just aren't enough hours in the day to do it all. The usual reaction to this "too much to do and not enough time" dilemma is to stop doing what God has called us to do and fall back into self-destructive behavior patterns. Wisdom suggests another option: When we find ourselves in "not enough time" mode, we need to immediately step back and assess our time priorities and make sure they align with God's priorities for our life.

For most, time is our most valuable resource, mainly because time is a fixed commodity. God allots time communistically: We all have a limited but equal 24-hour-per-day time allowance. We get no more; we get no less. If we use up today's time ration doing trivial things, we have to wait until tomorrow to get a new supply. Yet all too often, in an attempt to stretch our allotted time budget, we try to live on borrowed time. When we do that, what usually gets shortchanged in the transaction is our relationship with God—and our self-care efforts.

Although we talk about time management, in reality we do not have the power to manage time. The clock keeps ticking, no matter how hard we try to slow it down—or race against it to the finish line. However, we can manage ourselves in relation to the 24 hours God gives us each day. We can discipline ourselves to manage our time in accordance with God's priorities rather than fill our days with too many activities at a very high cost—the cost of our physical, mental, emotional and spiritual well-being.

When we don't take time for important things like exercising, meal planning, recreation and enough sleep, we are the ones who pay the price. Worse yet, we are robbing God. The Bible asks that we give God our first fruits, not what is left at the end of the day when we are too tired to spend quality time with Him (see Exodus 23:19). He gave his best for us; He deserves our best in return.

Second Peter 1:3 tells us God's "divine power has given us everything we need for life and godliness." The "everything we need" includes enough time. We know that our relationship with God is very high on His priority list, as is our physical, mental, emotional and spiritual well-being. Therefore, we need to look at things we can eliminate so that we will have enough time to do the things that are important to our Lord and Master. We need to identify the time thieves that gobble up the minutes we could be using according to God's plan and purpose. That's what giving Christ first place is all about: letting the Word of God, not the way of the world, define our time priorities.

Perhaps one of the best places to begin establishing God-honoring time priorities is to ask ourselves the question, *What am I doing that someone else could do so that I will have the time to do the one thing only I can do: maintain my personal relationship with God and care for myself?* Are you doing chores your children could do? Are you micromanaging rather than allowing others to be responsible for their own affairs? Are you in one-way relationships where you do all the giving while someone else does the taking? This will take an honest assessment of your situation. Take a moment to ponder that question and write your answer below.

_____

_____

_____

_____

Next, begin to look at the time thieves that keep you from accomplishing your health and fitness goals. Likely suspects are computer games, hours spent in front of the television, phone conversations with friends who don't respect your time boundaries, and co-workers who expect you to do your work and solve their problems, too. Carefully examine your life. Much like you use the Live It Tracker to record your food and exercise, and a budget to track your spending, keep a time log for a week or so; this will quickly bring your time thieves to light.

King David, according to 2 Samuel 24:24, declared, "I will not sacrifice to the LORD my God burnt offerings that cost me nothing." And so it is with us when it comes to time commitments. Yes, letting go of some of the things that currently take up your time may feel like a costly sacrifice. Satan is a master at getting us to do what is good so that there is not enough time left to do what is best. What are you currently doing that is good but is not part of God's best for you?

_____

_____

_____

_____

_____

Another valuable question when it comes to using your time as God intends it to be used is to ask yourself several times throughout the day, *What is it time for? Is it time for quiet time with the Lord? Is it time for exercise, work or meal planning? Is it time to be still and listen for God's still, small voice? Is it time to take a deep breath or get a glass of water? Is it time to write that note of encouragement or to call the friend who is struggling with out-of-control eating?* When we ask ourselves, *What is it time for?* unwanted distractions will not knock us off track and keep us from accomplishing our goals.

After three short years here on Earth, Jesus was able to say to His Father, "I have brought you glory on earth by completing the work you gave me to do" (John 17:4). Yes, there were still hungry, hurting people; and there were still those in need of healing, people who had not come to believe Jesus was the Christ of God. The world was still in need of revival, but Jesus had completed all the work His Father had given Him to do. Our loving Lord has also given you all the time you need to accomplish the purpose He has for your life. We are called to be prudent managers of all His good gifts, especially the gift of time. When God is in charge of our day planner, there is always enough time to do what is important to Him.

how to handle temptation!

Have you ever thought that if only you were stronger or more holy, you wouldn't be tempted? Temptation takes place when we think about something or acknowledge that we want to do something that isn't God's best for us. One way we can define "temptation" is to say that it is the desire to have or to do something that we know we should avoid. Temptation is a natural part of being human. Although temptation by itself is not sin, it is the door through which we can enter into sin. But God has provided a plan to help us handle temptation. First Corinthians 10:12-13 provides five truths that explain the nature of temptation and how to turn from it:

> So, if you think you are standing firm, be careful that you don't fall! No temptation has seized you except what is common to man. And God is faithful; he will not let you be tempted beyond what you can bear. But when you are tempted, he will also provide a way out so that you can stand up under it.

The first truth is that the areas in which we are the most confident and think we've got all figured out—or think that we don't need to rely on God or other people for help—are usually the areas in which we need to be the most careful. When we feel confident in our own abilities and our own strength, we are the most vulnerable, because we may not recognize the warning signs of temptation.

David's actions described in 2 Samuel 11 are an example of this. In this chapter, we read that David decided that he was confident enough in his kingship that he didn't have to go off to lead the troops in war. When he found himself unable to sleep one night, he discovered a woman bathing on her roof, and he inquired about her.

This action of David illustrates the second truth about temptation; it is common to all humankind. *All of us* are going to experience temptation at some point in our life. Your temptation is not unique to you. Just like seeing a beautiful woman may be tempting to all men, it was tempting to David, the king of Israel.

The third truth about temptation is that God is faithful. When we focus on God's faithfulness, we are able to understand that a temptation does not have to lead to sin. In fact, God allows us to be tempted, but He won't let us be tempted beyond our ability to handle it.

The fourth truth is that when we are tempted, we have a choice to make. We can either give in to the temptation or we can resist it. Even though it may not seem like we have the power to choose, *God provides a way out*, which means that we always have another option.

Finally, the fifth truth is that we can trust that the way out of the temptation will allow us to *stand up under it*—we can make a choice that leads to righteousness and not to sin.

So how do we develop a strategy for overcoming temptation?

1. **Trust God that there is a way out of every temptation.** When we understand that we always have the choice to turn from our temptation, we are better equipped to take the steps necessary to overcome temptation on a regular basis.

2. **Express your desire to the Lord to overcome the temptation, and ask Him to reveal the way out.** You cannot overcome temptation in your own strength, but you can overcome it through the power of the Holy Spirit and the Word of God. Dependence on God for your strength is an act of humility and establishes your need for His help.

3. **Look for a way of escape.** If you are tempted by chocolate and you can hear the chocolate "calling" your name from the kitchen each night when you sit down to watch your favorite TV show, find an alternative. Eat something to satisfy your desire for something sweet and creamy—nonfat chocolate pudding, for example! Or come up with an alternative action, such as muting the commercials and reading over your favorite Bible verses that speak to you about God's faithfulness and His love for you.

4. **Identify the steps that lead to your stumbling.** Most of us don't fall into temptation in one swift move; instead, we allow ourselves to entertain thoughts that lead us into sin. For instance, we might justify having just one piece of chocolate by telling ourselves that we deserve it because we've had a bad day. We must learn to identify the rationalizations we use, and we must remind ourselves that they are not based in truth but are lies we allow ourselves to believe.

5. **Establish a line you will not cross.** The best place to draw a line is at the thought pattern that leads to your stumbling. For instance, if the thought of how bad your day was usually leads you to eat chocolate, then draw the line so that when you start thinking about your day, you will think of a positive aspect for every negative aspect you identify. After a time, try coming up with more positive aspects than negative ones. Eventually, think of your day in terms of gratitude. Bad things may still happen, but you'll have a new way of thinking about them.

6. **Understand that there will be times when you may stumble.** We are most vulnerable to temptation when we are:

Hungry

Angry/**A**nxious

Lonely or

Tired (H.A.L.T.)

If you can identify the emotion, you can usually find an alternative to the temptation. However, there will be times when you will do the very thing you don't want to do. When this happens, it's common to feel guilty and ashamed, not to mention discouraged and disappointed in yourself. That's not what God desires for us, nor is it how He feels about us when we stumble. Romans 8:1 tells us that "there is now no condemnation for those of us who are in [relationship with] Christ Jesus." Instead, God provides us with His forgiveness, mercy and grace.

God's grace is the key element to this process of turning from temptation. When we understand how deeply God loves us and cheers us on toward success, and how He has provided Jesus' righteousness as our source of strength, we are empowered to overcome temptation in ways that we do not understand. When we choose to receive God's mercy and grace, we know that we are not on this journey alone. God is with us, and He will provide a way for us to overcome any temptation we face.

overcoming strongholds

D o you have a habit that you just can't seem to overcome no matter what you do and no matter how hard you try? The habit can be hidden or out in the open. It can be a destructive thought pattern or a behavior such as overspending, over-eating . . . over-anything. This habit may have such a hold on you that it controls your thoughts, your behaviors and maybe even your relationships. Something this pervasive and difficult to overcome is called a stronghold, because it has a very *strong hold* on your life.

HOW A STRONGHOLD STARTS

A stronghold usually has its start with a need to protect yourself from something—from a person or an emotion. In order to avoid the person or emotion, you turn to food. You eat something that makes you feel better momentarily and then you begin to associate feeling better with eating (or whatever you have done to feel better). It's not long before you eat whenever you don't feel your best. You eat when you're sad, lonely, stressed or bored. Then you eat in response to every emotion—even the positive ones—and you realize that you can't stop eating. When you try to diet or eat less, you don't know how to deal with the emotions that are still there. So you go back to eating.

Whenever an attitude or behavior begins to occupy a place of highest importance within you—even a good attitude or behavior—and you no longer have control over it, a stronghold is the result. In order to effectively deal with strongholds and get free from them, we first need to understand how strongholds are formed.

Thoughts
Strongholds have their root in the mind. The formation of a stronghold first starts when we allow ourselves to think or believe something contrary to what God says is true. When we think something that isn't consistent with what God tells us about Himself or about who

we are in Christ, we entertain a lie. When we're feeling down, the thought might be something as simple as, *A piece of cake would make me feel better,* or, *I need a new dress, even though I can't afford it.* Regardless of the thought, what we're doing is depending on something other than God to be the solution to a problem or challenge.

Emotions

Thoughts lead to emotions. When we feel a strong emotion, whether positive or negative, we can understand the emotion's presence by evaluating the thought that came to mind right before feeling the emotion. For instance, if you see flashing blue lights in your mirror, and you think, *Oh no, I'm speeding!* you're likely to experience a rush of anxiety. You would feel a very different emotion if you thought, *Good! They finally got here!*

Actions

Thoughts and emotions lead to action. We take action to resolve our emotions. Sometimes, however, our actions aren't positive. For instance, in the example just shared, if you were speeding, you could decide to make matters worse by leading the patrol car on a chase. Similarly, if you're feeling bored, scared or tense, you might decide to stuff your emotions with food or avoid your feelings by shopping. Conversely, it's entirely possible to allow a strong emotion to lead you toward a positive action. That's what First Place 4 Health will help you do.

Habits/Strongholds

Performing a specific action enough times will turn it into a habit. It's important to construct a positive action to break the destructive habit. For example, instead of always reaching for food to address negative feelings, you might use exercise as a way to cope with your emotions, which isn't a bad way to work through a problem. The caution here is not to let exercise (or anything else) become a stronghold by depending on it rather than God to balance your life. We know that we have a stronghold in our life when we depend on something and habitually seek that activity or thing instead of God to overcome the situation we wish to change.

HOW TO GET FREE FROM A STRONGHOLD

To overcome a stronghold, you have to evaluate the process you went through to establish the stronghold. Start by asking yourself some key questions that will help you determine why you took a particular action in response to a negative emotion.

1. *What is my stronghold/habit?* Does your habit draw you closer to God or keep you from experiencing the life He intends for you? Is the habit life-giving or life-taking?

2. *How did the habit get started?* Was it a coping mechanism for avoiding something negative? Was it a way to get through a difficult situation?

3. ***What emotions are associated with the stronghold?*** In order to truly overcome a stronghold, you have to visit the emotional level of the stronghold and identify the emotions that you might be trying to avoid.

4. ***What is the thought that results in that emotion?*** Strongholds are almost always based on deception. Maybe you grew up believing that you were not lovable, and you're afraid that if you allow yourself to be thin enough to attract attention, you will experience nothing but rejection, because nobody could ever love somebody like you.

Regardless of the thought, God gives us a strategy for dealing with strongholds:

> For though we live in the world, we do not wage war as the world does. The weapons we fight with are not the weapons of the world. On the contrary, they have divine power to demolish strongholds. We demolish arguments and every pretension that sets itself up against the knowledge of God, and we take captive every thought to make it obedient to Christ (2 Corinthians 10:3-5).

Paul tells us that the process is "to take captive every thought to make it obedient to Christ." This means that we challenge our irrational thoughts about who we are and what we need and compare them with the truth of God's Word. We choose to believe what God tells us. Here are a few thoughts you might want to challenge with God's truth:

The lie: *I'm not lovable.*

The truth: *"But God demonstrates his own love for us in this: While we were still sinners, Christ died for us"* (Romans 5:8).

The lie: *I'm a failure.*

The truth: *"Your hand will be lifted up in triumph over your enemies, and all your foes will be destroyed"* (Micah 5:9).

The lie: *I'll never change.*

The truth: *"Therefore, if anyone is in Christ, he is a new creation; the old has gone, the new has come!"* (2 Corinthians 5:17).

As you take your thoughts captive and challenge with the truth of God's Word the lies you have believed, you will begin to break down the stronghold that has controlled you. Each time you choose to believe God's Word, your need to seek something other than God to comfort or fill you will diminish until you are able to stop seeking things that lead you away from the good life God has always intended for you to live.

Remember that we are not to attempt to overcome a stronghold through worldly means. For example, we don't overcome a food stronghold through the latest fad diet or diet pills. We are to rely on God's power to change our thoughts, which will change our actions and demolish our strongholds.

GOD IS OUR STRONGHOLD

No one starts out thinking that he or she wants to be controlled by something—food or alcohol or negative self-talk. Dependence on those things sneaks up on us, and over time we become so attached to "that thing we do to cope" that we can't get free from it. But there is one expression of the word "stronghold" that not only is something to desire but also is something that brings great comfort and victory to our life. Psalm 144:2 tells us that God is our stronghold:

He is my loving God and my fortress, my stronghold and my deliverer, my shield, in whom I take refuge.

Who wouldn't want that kind of security?

Emotions

LEARN IT

- Accept the fact that both encouragement and accountability are necessary.
- Encourage others and encourage yourself.
- Build emotionally healthy relationships because they support positive change.
- Acknowledge that emotional control is part of total health.
- Eat for nutrition, not emotional numbness.
- Admit that change is a process, not an event.

LIVE IT

- Make accountability and encouragement a First Place 4 Health priority.
- Practice emotional satisfaction apart from food.
- Travel with friends (the role of encouragement and accountability).
- Choose specific strategies for positive change.
- Leave your past in the past.

the need for accountability and support

Two are better than one . . .
If one falls down, his friend can help him up. . . .
A cord of three strands is not quickly broken.

ECCLESIASTES 4:9-12

When we seek to change things in our life, a support system can help us make those changes faster and more thoroughly than if we live in isolation. It is a well-known fact that when we're connected to other people, we receive the support we need to persevere through life's struggles. Surrounded by supportive others, we are less likely to experience stress from our circumstances, become ill in the midst of our struggles or suffer from depression. When we're down or struggling with something, we need other people to encourage and help us; and encouragement is one way our support system helps us get through tough times. Another benefit of being part of a support system is accountability. Having people who will speak the truth to us in love helps us break through denial and face reality. Their love allows us to learn to embrace and accept both our strengths and our weaknesses.

That's why encouragement and accountability are the two most important functions of your First Place 4 Health group. The other members of your group will pray with and for you; they will share their joys and struggles and listen to yours, too. Because each First Place 4 Health group is made up of newcomers and those who have been in the program for many years, there will always be someone in your group who can minister to you, no matter what your need.

First Place 4 Health groups are arranged by divine appointment. Our sovereign and all-knowing God has intentionally put us in with other men and women with whom He knows we need to interact. Each person in your First Place 4 Health group is an important part of your change process, and you are a part of theirs. Although we have different backgrounds and personalities, we all share a common bond. By design, First Place 4 Health groups are made up of men and women who are striving to put Christ first in all things and who recognize that together we can do what none of us could do alone.

There are many benefits to having a healthy support system, but the greatest benefit is that when you're facing a challenge, you will have people who can lift you up in prayer, walk closely with you through your experience, and provide strength when you are weak.

what your first place 4 health group needs from you!

C ommunication is an essential part of any healthy relationship. If you can communicate effectively, you are on your way to a successful relationship. It is important that the members of your First Place 4 Health group clearly understand the role they are to play in your wellness journey and that you clearly understand the role you will play, too. Here are some specific ideas for effective group communication:

- **Be specific about the ways your group can help you.** Do not expect others to read your mind. If you need praise when you do well but not when you don't, tell your group. The more specific you are, the better your group will be able to help and encourage you. "Walk with me three mornings a week" is a much better request than "Encourage me to exercise."

- **Be honest with your group members.** Share your areas of weakness as well as your strengths. When you are willing to be vulnerable, the others in your group are encouraged to be vulnerable, too.

- **Be an encouragement to the others in your group.** A one-way relationship is never successful. Taking time to thank your group for their friendship, concern and support goes a long way in blessing your First Place 4 Health group for being a blessing to you.

- **Be trustworthy when handling prayer requests and concerns shared within your First Place 4 Health group.** Do not share information discussed within the group with those outside the group unless you have specific permission to do so. Confidentiality allows people to share their concerns, weaknesses and failures because they are confident that what is said in the group will stay in the group.

- **Be available when others in your group need your encouragement and support.** Availability begins with weekly attendance at First Place 4 Health group meetings and extends to the others things you do to attend to the others in your group on a daily basis.

- **Be active.** Remember, you will reap what you sow when it comes to group participation. If you want your group to be a source of support and encouragement for you, you will need to first do your part through active participation.

Ultimately, we are accountable to God and responsible for the choices we make. Hebrews 12:1 tells us to "throw off everything that hinders and the sin that so easily entangles, and let us run with perseverance the race marked out for us." We must run our own race to wellness, but a support network can be the tipping point that provides the strength and encouragement we need to make it to the finish line.

CHOOSING KEY ACCOUNTABILITY PARTNERS

When you establish a network of support, it's also important to identify one or two key people who can provide accountability apart from the group. These people should be part of your established support network, but will provide additional encouragement and responsibility for a specific change and a specified period of time. When you establish your accountability partners, keep in mind several things you must also choose to do:

- **Allow these individuals to ask you questions that will keep you focused on your goals.** You may feel vulnerable, but allowing your accountability partners to probe your thoughts and actions will help you identify areas of weakness before they become temptations or stumbling blocks.

- **Commit to honesty.** Your success in making healthy lifestyle changes is directly related to your willingness to openly and honestly share your struggles with your accountability partners.

- **Commit to seeking input prior to taking action.** If you talk to your accountability partners prior to making decisions or taking action, you will have the opportunity to consider other points of view before you move in a specific direction. A commitment to ask for input will help you learn what to consider as you make important decisions.

- **Strive for internal accountability.** As you make the changes for which you have sought accountability, you will begin to develop the ability to process decisions and avoid temptations on your own. There will come a time when your internal accountability system includes prayer, relying on God for direction, commitment to following Him and His Word, and the ability to hold yourself accountable. Once you do this on a consistent basis, you probably won't need external accountability and can release your partners from their responsibility. It's important to involve your accountability partners in this decision so that you do not release them prematurely.

Establishing a support system may take time, but the reward is that you will experience a sense of belonging, security and encouragement as you face challenges and start making changes that will help you live the life God intends for you to live.

intentional acts of encouragement!

*Encourage one another daily, . . . so that none of you
may be hardened by sin's deceitfulness.*

HEBREWS 3:13

Encouragement is an intentional act intended to infuse another with renewed courage, renewed hope and renewed strength. As the word "encourage" tells us, this intentional act fills those who are weak or faltering in their faith with the courage to persevere, especially in times of trial. In Hebrews 3:13, "encouragement" is translated from a Greek word that was used when fearful, hesitant, fainthearted soldiers and sailors were sent into battle. In First Place 4 Health, intentional acts of encouragement serve the same purpose. Although we aren't going into a physical battle against a visible enemy, we are engaged in a fierce spiritual battle as we strive to overcome the forces that threaten to keep us in defeat and despair.

In 1 Thessalonians 5:11, Paul tells us to "encourage one another and build each other up." Encouragement is a ministry that every member of a First Place 4 Health group is called to develop and practice. Each such act that we do is an intentional act of encouragement, because unless we are deliberate in our efforts, we will not be faithful encouragers. Our best intentions will not get the card mailed, the email sent, the phone call made. Like most of the other actions we take in First Place 4 Health, we need to be mindful and purposeful in our encouragement of the others in our First Place 4 Health group. There are at least four reasons why we need to take our responsibility as encouragers very seriously:

1. *Encouragement is an urgent need for those who are trying to overcome negative habits, or patterns of behavior.* In Hebrews 3: 13, we are told to "encourage one another daily, . . . so that none of [us] may be hardened by sin's deceitfulness." The world we live in is full of things that pull us

down. As people striving to break free of the destructive behavior patterns that characterized our past, we urgently need others who will lift us up with intentional acts of encouragement.

2. *Encouragement is the unique priority of the God we serve.* Throughout the pages of Scripture, each member of the Trinity (God the Father, God the Son and God the Holy Spirit) serves as an encourager. God the Father is described as "the Father of compassion" (2 Corinthians 1:3). Even in the final moments of His life on Earth, Jesus the Son comforted and encouraged His fearful disciples. And encouragement is implied by one of the Holy Spirit's names! Paraclete, or Holy Spirit, is translated from the Greek word *parakletos,* which means advocate or counselor. So when we encourage people, we live out the ministry of the third Person of the Trinity. God the Father encourages. God the Son encourages. God the Holy Spirit encourages. As Christians we need to be encouragers because encouragement is a primary ministry, a priority, of our triune God.

3. *Encouragement is one of God's purposes in giving us the Bible.* Paul tells us that "everyone who prophesies [speaks the word of God] speaks to men for their strengthening, encouragement and comfort" (1 Corinthians 14:3). In Romans 15, Paul reminds us that one of the purposes of the Old Testament was to provide encouragement for us today. "For everything that was written in the past was written to teach us, so that through endurance and the encouragement of the Scriptures we might have hope" (Romans 15:4). Scripture was written by the God of hope to infuse us with strength and courage. As Christ followers, it is our responsibility to use the Word of God to encourage others who need to be built up in their faith.

4. *Encouragement is infectious.* Picture a pebble thrown into water. At first there is an immediate impact, and then the ripples continue indefinitely. That's what an intentional act of encouragement is like—it begins a never-ending process. Having been encouraged, our first reaction is to encourage someone else. Encouragement begins a process that goes on forever as each intentional act of encouragement builds up others in their faith; and they, in turn, pass on the encouragement to others in need of strength, comfort and endurance.

Each week you will be asked to intentionally encourage the other members of your First Place 4 Health group. At other times, the Holy Spirit will bring a member of your group to mind, perhaps in answer to that person's prayers for help. Your responsibility as an encourager is to be faithful to your calling, which is to encourage one another daily. When it comes to offering encouragement, there is no better way to infuse another with courage than to use the very words of Scripture. You might want to include the week's memory verse in your phone calls, emails, cards and face-to-face conversations. The Holy Spirit might bring a different verse to mind as you talk to someone who is struggling. Being able to recall the exact verse that another needs in a time of trouble is a wonderful benefit of Scripture memory!

In addition to the blessings others receive when you are faithful to do intentional acts of encouragement, as a faithful encourager you will be built up in your own faith. As you write or say the words of Scripture to another, you take them in, too! Often, in the providence of God, He sends people for us to encourage because He knows we need to hear the words we will say to them. In a word full of lose-lose situations, encouragement is a win-win proposition!

Finally, be sure not to confuse encouragement and flattery. Flattery is intended to puff up; encouragement is given to build up. Flattery keeps us from facing the truth of our situation so that we can take appropriate action. Encouragement tells the truth in love. Here are some tips to help you become a faithful First Place 4 Health intentional encourager:

- Write down the phone number of every member of your First Place 4 Health group and keep the list by your phone, or program the list into your cell phone's address book.

- Put your First Place 4 Health group roster on your computer desk top, and/or place a copy in your prayer journal.

- Carry a small packet of note cards with you to appointments where you know you will have some wait time. As you wait, you can fill your time by writing words of encouragement to a group member.

- Write "time for encouragement" on your daily calendar.

- Place some note cards in your quiet-time space so that as the Holy Spirit brings group members to mind, you can be instantly obedient to His encouragement to encourage others.

- Put a note on your refrigerator to remind you to be an encourager, not an overeater.

- Make your encouragement simple and specific. Rather than simply forwarding group emails to others, write your own personal words of encouragement.

- Remember that encouragers are listeners, not just talkers!

- Rather than agreeing to add someone to your personal prayer list, pray with that person immediately—either in person or over the phone.

emotionally healthy
relationships

We were created for relationship—with God and with people. In fact, the Bible tells us that the greatest commandment is to *love God* and *love people* (see Luke 10:27). If we were created for relationship and God's Word tells us that loving Him and loving others is His will for us, then why is it so difficult sometimes to develop personal relationships that thrive and flourish?

Part of the challenge is that we invite into our inner circle of trusted relationships the wrong people or those who are not yet ready to be included. When their behavior doesn't resemble that of a trusted friend, we tend to react in one of two ways: (1) we shut down and refuse entrance to the person who has betrayed our trust, or (2) we continue to suffer disappointment and hurt by letting the person remain privy to our hearts. The issue here isn't whether we should shut down and evict people from our lives; the issue is that we need to carefully assess each friendship for what it is and act accordingly.

ASSESSMENT OF FRIENDS

How can you wisely assess how to invite people into your inner circle of trust? In the book *Safe People: How to Find Relationships That Are Good for You and Avoid Those That Aren't*, authors Henry Cloud and John Townsend indicate that safe relationships (1) draw us closer to God, (2) draw us closer to others, and (3) help us become the real person God created us to be.[1]

Closer to God

A trusted friend shows love for God and a desire to seek Him. God's commandment, recorded in Luke 10:27, is to "'love the Lord your God with all of your heart and with all your soul and with all your strength and with all your mind'; and, 'Love your neighbor as yourself.'" Therefore, it's important that our friendships be characterized by love for the Lord. As we grow closer to people, we need to be sure that they are helping us draw closer to God and that we are helping them draw closer to Him.

Closer to Others

A trusted friend is one who cares about good communication. This includes both the ability to share at a level that goes below the surface and the ability to truly listen. A healthy relationship allows you to share your true feelings in a safe environment. James 1:19 tells us that we should make listening a priority—we "should be quick to listen, slow to speak and slow to become angry." If each person in a relationship is more focused on listening instead of talking, communication patterns will take on a healthy balance.

Closer to Being the Real Person God Created You to Be

Inner-circle friends create a trust that brings out the best in you. Trust comes from having a mutual respect for what is best in each other's lives. When we know that someone is truly concerned about us, we are more likely to trust what the person is saying and to continue to invest in the relationship. Trust makes it possible to disagree or share constructive feedback without either person taking offense. Healthy relationships make it possible for disagreements to lead to relationship growth.

This may seem paradoxical, but *inner-circle friends set and respect boundaries in the relationship.* Often we have a hard time saying no to our friends. A mark of health in a friendship is being able to say no at appropriate times without experiencing a negative impact on the relationship. This includes not jumping to the rescue each time a friend has a need but, instead, turning to the Lord in prayer on the friend's behalf and allowing the Lord to meet the person's needs. When a relationship is healthy, both parties understand the boundaries that exist for the other person, and they respect the other's right to establish such boundaries.

If someone doesn't exhibit these characteristics, you have to ask yourself if the friendship is safe and trustworthy.

CIRCLE OF FRIENDS

Take some time to think about your friendships, and picture them as existing within one of four circles that get smaller toward the center (similar to a bull's-eye).

Circle One

The innermost circle includes the people who demonstrate the healthiest aspects of friendship. These people are the ones with whom you will share your deepest feelings, thoughts and desires. They are the individuals who will influence you the most and with whom you will have the most influence. This circle should include your spouse, possibly other family members and only a few other trusted friends.

Proverbs 18:24 addresses this level of friendship: "A man of many companions may come to ruin, but there is a friend who sticks closer than a brother." Because you are allowing the individuals in this circle to influence you, it is important that these people have a strong and growing relationship with the Lord. Biblical examples of inner-circle friendships can be found in the friendship between David and Jonathan (see 1 Samuel 20:42) and between Mary and Elizabeth (see Luke 1:39-56).

Circle Two

The second circle includes those people with whom you share some of your feelings, thoughts and desires, but not all of them. They are people who have some influence over you, and you have some influence over them. You would consider their counsel, but may not automatically accept it. This level of friendship may include people you are mentoring or encouraging to develop a stronger relationship with God.

Circle Three

The third circle includes people you don't know as well as those in Circles One and Two. You may interact with these people because you share common interests or stage-of-life circumstances. People in this circle are folks you might engage in a conversation about your faith, but you may not readily know if they have a relationship with the Lord. You might spend time with these people to influence them to know the Lord, but you are unlikely to be influenced by them because they do not share the same desire as you do to know the Lord in an ever-deepening way.

Circle Four

The outer circle includes people with whom you interact on an occasional basis. Maybe they are people you run into at sporting events or the library. You do not influence these people in a significant way, and they don't have the opportunity to influence you. You might share cordial greetings and know their names, but you don't seek them out for support or encouragement.

It's possible for people to move from one circle to another, depending on what is happening in the individual's life or in your life. By understanding what makes a healthy relationship, you are able to make wise decisions about who belongs in which circle of friends and when it is safe to allow someone into a closer friendship with you.

Now that you have a better idea of why some people feel safe and others feel less so, look at your own behavior and consider how you could become a better friend to those few people who are in your inner circle of trust. Fill in, where appropriate, the names of people you're friends with, and, where appropriate, tell an issue that would need a boundary set.

CHARACTERISTICS OF AN UNHEALTHY RELATIONSHIP

- Controlling or manipulative behavior on either side

- Guilt about the things you do to establish boundaries in the relationship

- Frequent negative feelings when you are around the person

- Fulfilling one person's needs at the expense of the other's needs

- Lies, secrets or a legitimate lack of trust

My inner-circle relationships are with _____
_____
_____ .

_____ encourages me to draw closer to God.

I could influence _____ to trust God
more if _____ .

_____ listens to me as much as she talks.

I could talk less and listen more to _____ .

I could show more respect to _____ by
setting a boundary around the issue of _____
_____ .

I could ask for more respect from _____ by
setting a boundary around the issue of _____
_____
_____ .

Based on the principles of loving God first, practicing good communication and
showing themselves worthy of trust, which people in Circles Two, Three or Four
might be ready to move closer to or into your inner circle of relationships?

_____
_____
_____
_____
_____
_____
_____
_____

Note

1. Henry Cloud and John Townsend, *Safe People: How to Find Relationships That Are Good for You and Avoid Those That Aren't* (Grand Rapids, MI: Zondervan Publishing House, 1996), p. 143.

you and your emotions

When God created us, He gave us the capacity to feel emotions. As early as the Garden of Eden, we can see that our emotions are an innate part of who we are. When God asked Adam, "Where are you?" Adam told Him that he was afraid, so he hid (see Genesis 3:9-10). There are many other Scripture passages that denote the legitimacy of emotions. For example, we are told to "rejoice with those who rejoice; mourn with those who mourn" (Romans 12:15).

Even when we are convinced that the ability to feel a variety of emotions is a good thing, we often label our emotions as either good or bad. When we feel joy, that's a good thing. When we feel sad, that's a bad thing. Emotions, however, are neither good nor bad. They are neutral, and they serve an important purpose in our life.

Throughout the New Testament, we find examples of how Jesus demonstrated a vast range of emotions. He felt compassion; He was zealous, angry, deeply moved, indignant, troubled, full of joy; He was very sorrowful, greatly distressed, depressed and grieved. As children of God, we have the freedom to demonstrate the same full range of emotions that we see in Jesus. Our challenge is to demonstrate them *in the appropriate manner* and *at the appropriate time* and *directed toward the appropriate person or situation*.

IN THE APPROPRIATE MANNER

We often connect emotions with memories. For instance, if you have fond childhood memories of your father (or mother) walking in the house and announcing, "I'm home!" you will feel a positive emotion when you hear a family member say the same thing. If your memory is attached to anxiety (perhaps your father or mother was an angry person), then you might cringe when you hear a family member announce his or her arrival. Responding in an appropriate manner involves separating your past memories from the current situation and not letting your memories rule your emotions.

AT THE APPROPRIATE TIME

Often we store up our negative reactions. When we finally do express them, they spew onto the people around us. We need to learn to express our emotions when we experience them. When Jesus saw the money handlers and animal merchants in his Father's house, He was angry, and He demonstrated His anger by turning the tables over and telling them all to leave (see John 2:14-15). He didn't wait until the next time he saw the same situation, and He didn't store up the injustices He saw and blast the people later. He spoke truth in the moment.

However, a word of caution is necessary here: We sometimes allow our emotions to consume us, and the appropriate time to express our emotions may not be in the moment. That's when it's important to tell the person you're talking with that you need to wait until you can calm down before you can talk through what you're feeling. Then you need to follow up with the person once you have had time to process and pray through your feelings.

TOWARD THE APPROPRIATE PERSON OR SITUATION

When we feel something unpleasant that we don't want to express, we might transfer what we're feeling toward one person or situation onto another person or situation. For example, if you find out that your job is being eliminated, you might then go home and yell at your children. Jesus demonstrated for us how to handle this type of situation. When He was asleep in the boat and His followers woke Him up because of the storm, instead of rebuking the disciples for waking Him up, He "rebuked the wind" and told the waves to be calm (Mark 4:39). We need to think through why we are feeling what we're feeling so that we can direct our feelings toward the appropriate person or situation.

Here are three principles to remember when it comes to understanding our emotions:

1. *We were not created for our emotions; our emotions were created for us.* We were not created to be ruled by our emotions and to allow our emotions to damage our lives and our relationships. Instead, God gave us emotions so that we can identify our values and what is important to us. When we cry because someone we know is hurting, we are expressing the value of that relationship. Our emotions were created to help us understand what is important in our lives.

2. *Emotions are a barometer of our soul.* Emotions allow us to identify when something doesn't line up with what we believe or think. Experiencing a strong negative emotion is an indicator that something isn't resting well in our heart. The challenge is to use that emotion to explore what is wrong and to work with God to resolve the imbalance.

3. *We can have emotional control.* Even though we have a long history of being controlled by our emotions, emotional balance is still possible. Whether we manage or mismanage our emotions, as we take them to the Lord, He will help us develop self-control and learn to rely on the Holy Spirit to achieve the appropriate emotional responses to the situations we face.

handling your emotions so that they don't handle you!

A commonly held misconception about life after becoming a Christian is that there will be no more problems, no more pain, no more mess-ups. Along with that general mindset is the thought that growing in Christ will permanently prevent the need to deal with negative emotions. Have you ever thought, for example, that because you are a Christian, you should never get angry, only to discover that life can include acute disappointments and discouragements? It's easy to assume that if we're walking closely with the Lord, we won't experience painful emotions. The reality of daily life, however, often includes situations that result in emotional pain or even trauma, so we need to learn how to handle those feelings before they handle us.

One important reason to learn to manage your emotions is because uncontrolled negative emotions can provide Satan a foothold in your life. Scripture instructs us to give our burdens to God instead of holding on to them: "Cast all your anxiety on him because he cares for you. Be self-controlled and alert. Your enemy the devil prowls around like a roaring lion looking for someone to devour" (1 Peter 5:7-8). What a great prescription for getting out from under negative emotions and dodging the attacks of our enemy: We simply need to place them in God's care!

Being self-controlled when it comes to handling our emotions isn't always an easy thing to do. Most of us respond to our emotions in one of three ways:

1 We suppress them.

2 We overexpress them.

3 We appropriately recognize them.

Suppression involves pushing your feelings down or denying they exist. Have you ever tried to ignore your feelings or chosen not to deal with them? When you do this, you basically deny that you feel anything. If you suppress your feelings long enough, you might find it difficult to even know what you feel, whether the feelings are positive or negative. Since negative emotions are an indicator that something isn't right in your heart, suppressing emotions can be dangerous and keep you from acknowledging that you're in danger in some way or keep you from creating healthy boundaries in your life. Suppressing emotions can also keep you from having a healthy relationship with God and with other people. In Psalm 39, David spoke of his increased anguish when he kept silent.

Overexpression of emotions happens when you decide to tell everyone around you exactly how you feel. Some people call this venting, but it usually goes beyond a need to let off steam and results in casting your burdens on other people through outbursts that can destroy relationships. Overexpressing your emotions often leads you to say things you don't mean.

Appropriate recognition of emotions is the process of being honest about how you feel—first with God and then with a few trusted friends. As you learn to take your hurt and anger to God and to those who love you unconditionally, you will be less likely to let your feelings affect your relationships. God is not surprised or shocked by any of your feelings, regardless of how vile they may seem to you. In Psalm 109:6-20, David cried out to God for God to punish David's enemies, to make David's enemies suffer great consequences. Still, God called David "a man after [God's] own heart" (Acts 13:22).

To be able to move from an unhealthy way of expressing your feelings to a more appropriate way, you must understand where your feelings come from. For the most part, feelings are the emotional reaction you have to your thoughts. Remember the earlier example of seeing flashing blue lights in your car's rearview mirror, which almost always evokes an emotional response? What you think will determine whether the flashing lights will trigger anxiety or relief. Therefore, it's important to evaluate what thoughts precede your strong emotions if you are going to succeed in handling your emotions before they handle you.

Often there is a thought *pattern* that negatively affects your emotions. If you can learn to take your thoughts captive to the truth of Christ (see 2 Corinthians 10:5), you can learn to handle your emotions in a healthy manner. Beliefs or thought patterns that have been reinforced by what others have said about you, by your own view of your competence or by your own negative thoughts can be reframed and your thinking transformed through Scripture. For example, you might be depressed because you believe you will never be successful at reaching the fitness level you desire. Maybe as a child you heard over and over again that you were fat, and that experience has played out in your history of not being successful at your fitness goals. You can now choose, however, to believe what God's Word tells

THE THREE WAYS TO HANDLE EMOTIONS

- *Suppression* involves pushing your feelings down or denying they exist.

- *Over-expression* of emotions happens when you decide to tell everyone around you exactly how you feel.

- *Appropriate recognition* of emotions is the process of being honest about how you feel—first with God and then with a few trusted friends.

you in Philippians 4:13: "I can do everything through [Christ] who gives me strength" and over time live in the light of this truth.

Additionally, it's important to realize that your unhealthy emotions may be an indicator of a deeper emotional need that has resulted from trauma. People who habitually either suppress or over-express their emotions often find that they have developed this strategy as a coping mechanism for something they were not able to deal with appropriately when it happened. If you identify that your expression of emotions is a way to avoid feelings or is the result of feelings that you haven't been able to handle, you may want to seek a trusted Christian counselor who will walk with you through the process of identifying the source of those emotions and help you experience God's healing in your heart.

stress-related eating!

One of the clearest definitions of "stress" is "resistance to what is." We feel stress when we are unable to make happen what we want or need to happen, given the circumstances we're facing. Sometimes we overeat because we want something comforting in an uncomfortable situation; sometimes we just want something quick and convenient in a busy day, and we end up making the wrong food choices. Regardless of the reason, what we pack in during moments of stress packs on the pounds.

Here are some physical, psychological and behavioral warning signs that indicate that you are feeling overly burdened by life's circumstances, which can tempt you to throw out your good intentions to choose quality food in the proper quantities:

- Headache, indigestion, fatigue, sleeplessness, high blood pressure, frequent illness (physical)

- Depression, anger, hypersensitivity, fuzzy thinking, irritability, anxiety (psychological)

- Increased appetite or loss of appetite, procrastination, poor job performance, impatience, isolation, burnout (behavioral)

What can you do to alleviate stress-related eating? The first and best strategy is to turn to your guidebook for life—the Bible. Jesus said in Matthew 11:28, "Come to me, all you who are weary and burdened, and I will give you rest." Notice that He didn't tell us to manage our time better or to stop procrastinating so much. He said that when we feel stressed or burdened, we should come to Him and let Him give us His peace and carry our burden on His shoulders.

In addition to giving our stressful burdens to Jesus, there are some other things we can do. An effective physical strategy for managing stress is to get moving. It's a common misconception to think that we're too busy or too tired to exercise. While exercise does take energy, in the long run, it produces energy. Exercise actually increases brain-cell growth in the part of the brain that is responsible for controlling stress, so consistent exercise has a major impact on our ability to manage stress over time.

Another strategy is to practice relaxation techniques, such as deep breathing. Once your mind is more relaxed, you can think about what is causing your stress and if it's serious enough to require all the emotional energy you're focusing on the situation.

And then there's the importance of down time. Do you need to address aspects of your life that leave no discretionary time to recharge? When you're constantly on the go, you don't have the opportunity to rejuvenate and process what's going on in your life. Even God rested after creating the world and everything in it—not because He needed to rest but because it was an important part of evaluating all that He had done (see Genesis 2:2-3).

Although we can't change the reality that we will feel pressured at times—by family, job, finances, illness, or any number of other things—we can learn to manage our reaction to the common stresses of life.

TIPS TO HELP YOU AVOID STRESS-RELATED EATING

1. If you can't get food out of your thoughts, drink something satisfying and wait 30 minutes. If the food craving passes, then you weren't really hungry.

2. If you typically snack at specific times of the day or after specific occasions, change your routine.

3. Write down what you eat on a daily basis so that you can identify if you overeat on any given stressful day. Awareness provides opportunity to change.

4. Don't combine eating with another activity, such as watching television or driving. Keeping activities separate will encourage you to be mindful about what you are eating.

5. If too many hours pass between meals or snacks, your blood sugar will plummet and you will be more likely to overeat. So eat before you get famished.

6. Every day, pray through your favorite Scripture verses about food, self-control and your body as a temple.

7. Identify the locations where you are most likely to eat when you're feeling stressed, and avoid those places on busy or chaotic days. If you usually eat while driving, chew some gum or sip a bottle of water or a noncaloric beverage.

8. Keep a daily record of what you eat, and review it before each meal. When you're aware of what you've already eaten that day, you may choose to forego that extra helping or sweet. Plus you will form the good habit of thinking before you eat.

9. If you have a pattern of snacking at a certain time of day, keep yourself occupied during that period.

10. Practice eating only when you're sitting down. This will allow you to savor your food.

If you're feeling a bit stressed just reading through these suggestions, remember two things: (1) God doesn't want you to be exhausted by your efforts to be less stressed, and (2) these strategies should not be regarded as more things for you to do. Think instead about the fact that you will reap what you sow. If you sow rest and retraining of your thoughts to deal with improper food consumption, over time you will reap the rewards of better health.

are you an emotional eater?

There's a famous song in the musical *Oliver* that includes the phrase "Food, glorious food!" That phrase has become a proclamation for many of us about the connection of food consumption with our emotions. Oliver, however, was an orphan boy dreaming of what a life of prosperity would be like, not someone looking for a way to deal with negative feelings.

Food gives us energy and provides health—and it's important to nourish our bodies. Unfortunately, many of us have made food consumption a way to cope with negative emotions—and sometimes even with positive ones. But that's not the role God intended food to play in our lives.

Ask yourself the following questions to determine if you use food to fill an emotional need:

1. *Do I sometimes put food in my mouth before I realize I've done it?*
2. *Does eating cause me to feel stressed or guilty?*
3. *When I get in a disagreement with someone or I'm bored, do I think of eating?*
4. *Do I eat more when I have a lot of time on my hands?*
5. *Have I developed a strategy for dealing with my emotions that doesn't involve eating?*
6. *Does eating something fattening early in the day negatively affect my food choices for the whole day?*
7. *Do I consider food my enemy?*
8. *Do I wander around thinking I want something to eat, but I don't know what it is?*
9. *Do I crave something to eat, even when I'm not hungry?*
10. *Do I sometimes snack to avoid doing something else I need to do?*

If you answered yes to most of the above questions, you're probably looking for something to munch on instead of dealing with something you're feeling. This is sometimes called thought hunger because it helps us avoid the emotions that come from the less-than-pleasant things we're thinking about.

If you have identified that you eat for emotional reasons, then you need to develop healthy alternatives to cope with your emotions. Fill in the blanks of these statements to discover things you can do instead of eating through your feelings.

- When I really want to relax, I _____.
  (Do this when you're overwhelmed or overly busy.)

- When I talk to _____, my problems don't seem so huge.
  (Talk to this person when you're hurt or angry.)

- I always laugh a lot when I spend time with _____.
  (Spend time with this person when you're sad or down about something.)

- The Scriptures that encourage me the most are_____

  _____.

  (Read these passages when you feel discouraged.)

- I love hanging out with _____.
  (Spend time with this person when you're feeling lonely.)

If you can't do any of these things, here are additional ideas for dealing with the desire to eat something when you're not hungry:

- Take a walk in your favorite park or neighborhood and really see the beauty of the landscape, the architecture of the houses, and the variety of plants and flowers.
- Take a long bubble bath.
- Play outside with your pet.
- Learn a new craft: beading, scrapbooking, model building—or whatever else catches your interest.
- Catch up with a friend by phone, or write an overdue thank-you note.
- Clean out a drawer in the kitchen or organize your garage.
- Invite a friend over for dinner.
- Volunteer to help someone run an errand, mow a lawn or do a simple home repair.
- Go to your local library, and take home a book to read.

When dealing with negative feelings, we need a list of alternatives that will redirect our attention. But we also need to seek God's help in managing our emotions and learning how to take our feelings to Him instead of to the refrigerator. He tells us in His Word that He "will meet all [our] needs according to his glorious riches in Christ Jesus" (Philippians 4:19) and that we have been enriched by Him in every way (see 1 Corinthians 1:5). He is our best source for receiving comfort and meeting our emotional needs. Instead of singing "Food, glorious food!" let's begin to sing "God, glorious God!"

mapping your emotional
history with food!

We were created for relationship with God and with people, but when those relationships fall short of what God intended them to be, there is a void in our heart. God, first of all, wants to fill that void with Himself. Second Corinthians 1:5 tells us, "For just as the sufferings of Christ flow over into our lives, so also through Christ our comfort overflows." The Holy Spirit, who is always with us, is available to comfort us when we are feeling lonely, sad, hurt, angry or whatever we feel that quenches our joy.

Many of us, however, have failed to find our comfort in the Lord and instead have sought fulfillment from food. God wants to fulfill our emotional needs with Himself and through other people, not with food.

As we identify the ways we have built an unhealthy relationship with food, God is waiting for us to turn our hearts back to Him. In Isaiah 61:1, we learn that Jesus came "to proclaim freedom for the captives, and release from darkness for the prisoners" (that's you and me). When we ask, He will reveal to us the patterns and habits that are so far away from the abundant life we desire and that He has promised to give us.

In order to experience that abundant life, we first have to identify the patterns we have developed and map out the role that food has played in keeping us from experiencing what was promised. Mapping our emotional history with food will help us evaluate each stage of our life (early childhood, childhood, teen years, college years, single years and married years) in order to discover the reasons behind why we struggle with food issues.

To map your emotional history with food, you will need paper and pen to record your thoughts and an extended period (or perhaps more than one extended period) of uninterrupted time. As you begin, ask God to bring to mind what you need to remember.

Step 1: Ask God for clarity to identify thoughts, emotions and patterns of behavior that have resulted in your current emotional relationship with food. As you pray, ask God to reveal truth to you through this process and allow you to visit the deep places of your heart to bring about inner wisdom (see Psalm 51:6).

Father, I know that You are the God of all wisdom, and right now I need wisdom about the relationship between my emotions and food . . .

Step 2: Label separate sheets of paper with each major stage of your life, starting with early childhood and ending with your current stage.

Early Childhood. Childhood. Teen Years. College Years. Single Years. Married Years.

Step 3: Think back to the earliest time in your life that you can remember and write out the story of what life was like for you during that period. Go as deep into your heart as you can, even if expressing those emotions is painful. The Lord will guide you to the memories and experiences that have impacted you the most. Jesus tells us that God sent Jesus "to comfort all who mourn . . . to bestow on them a crown of beauty instead of ashes, the oil of gladness instead of mourning, and a garment of praise instead of a spirit of despair" (Isaiah 61:2-3).

By the age of 6 or 7, home didn't feel safe anymore . . . I began to gain weight . . . food was comforting . . .

Step 4: Identify when there were major changes in your life and describe how you responded to those changes (such as a family move, graduation from high school, or marriage). Maybe you began eating more when your parents divorced, or you lost a significant amount of weight just before a major change in your life. Thoroughly explore the patterns of your eating behaviors and your weight during each of the periods you write about.

When I was 12, my family moved to a new state. It was hard to make friends. I didn't like the new area much . . .

Step 5: Be specific about your feelings, destructive patterns of behavior, choices and longings. At the same time, be sure to also include your strengths so that you develop a balanced view of your life and who you really are.

Food comforted me and made me feel good, and it also kept me away from the rejection I feared would come if I were thin . . .

Step 6: Ask God to help you remember what you may have forgotten or have blocked from your memory. Ask Him to reveal the true story of your life and the relationship you have developed with food.

Lord, show me if there is anything that I have forgotten or blocked from my memory. I desire to live in truth about my life . . .

Step 7: After you have reviewed and prayed through each of the stages, take some time to write down what you have discovered from this experience. Ask the Lord to show you the connection between your eating and your emotions, the events of your life and the patterns you have developed to cope with certain events, and the ways that food has kept you from becoming the person God desires you to be.

> *There is a connection between my weight and my relationships. When I fail at relationships, I turn to food to comfort me . . .*

Step 8: If you are able to see well-defined patterns and you are prepared to turn from the destructive behaviors you have developed, take some time to pray and make a commitment, both in prayer and in writing, to the changes God has led you to make.

> *Lord, I am committed to learning new ways of dealing with my emotions and not allowing failed relationships to lead me to destructive eating patterns . . .*

Step 9: Finally, write a prayer of repentance and rededication to God. Don't forget to thank Him for allowing you to search your heart so deeply and revealing the wounds He wants to heal in you. Thank Him for the work He is going to do in you as you turn back to Him and allow food to play its proper role—to bring physical nourishment to your body.

> *As of today . . . you are out of my life! I will eat for God's glory . . .*

Jesus promised, "If you hold to my teaching, you are really my disciples. Then you will know the truth, and the truth will set you free" (John 8:31-32). As you continue to seek Him in the process of returning food to its proper role in your life, you will find the freedom that results from the abundant life Jesus promised we would have.

the change process

Once you identify the need to change the role food plays in your life, it's time to develop strategies for change. It's important to change not only your behaviors but also your thoughts so that you can address the core issues that created the need for your unhealthy relationship with food.

"Change" is a word that causes many of us to feel uneasy. We like what is comfortable and familiar. That's one reason why we allow behaviors and habits that are inconsistent with our health goals to remain in our life.

It's true that the process of change can be uncomfortable, and change does take time. Unfortunately, when we don't see immediate results, we're often tempted to stop persevering through the change process. But change requires our focused attention, and we have to get used to new ways of thinking and behaving that are out of our comfort zone.

INTENTIONAL DISCOMFORT

Stand up and fold your arms in front of you. Now take the arm that is on top and place it underneath your other arm. How does that feel? If you're like most people, it feels a little off. Now open your arms and fold them again. Did you go back to the way you naturally fold your arms, or did you fold them the new (and probably uncomfortable) way?

The patterns and behaviors we develop over time, even if they are unhealthy, become difficult to change. The good news is that if we are willing to experience the discomfort of the change process, what was once uncomfortable for us will eventually become comfortable, and we will reap the benefits of a new intentional habit.

The process of change is much like the discipline process described in Hebrews 12:11: "No discipline seems pleasant at the time, but painful. Later on, however, it produces a harvest of righteousness and peace for those who have been trained by it." When we speak of discipline in this context, we are not referring to punishment or correction for wrongdoing; we are disciplining our lives for our good. In the moment, the process of change the Lord brings us through is uncomfortable; but in the end, it produces right living.

TRAINING FOR RIGHT LIVING

Because we reinforce our eating habits on a daily basis—making choices several times a day about what we are going to eat, how much we are going to eat and when we are going to eat— one of the most challenging change processes starts when we decide to change how we relate to food. How can you make needed changes when it comes to the role of food in your life?

1. *Ask the Lord about what needs to change.* You can't permanently change your behaviors or thoughts in regard to food without involving the Lord in the process. Ask Him to reveal to you how to eat for His glory (see 1 Corinthians 10:31). To determine what changes are necessary, ask Him to help you assess how much you eat, what types of food you regularly consume and how often you eat.

2. *Keep track of food consumption for a week to determine your current eating habits.* After you read through your food record, go back to the Lord in prayer, and ask Him to show you specific ways you can change your eating habits to effectively care for His temple (see 1 Corinthians 6:19). If He shows you several changes to make, try to prioritize those changes, based on how important they are to your overall success.

3. *Pick one change to implement this week.* Focus on the new behavior for a period of at least one week.

4. *As you become more comfortable with each new behavior, continue to identify changes to implement from your priority list.* Don't try to change all behaviors at the same time or they may turn out to be only temporary changes. For lifelong change to take place, you must intentionally work the change into your life until it becomes a comfortable habit.

5. *Spend time in prayer, evaluating how you're doing with the changes you're practicing.* Ask the Lord to continue to identify how you can make healthy habits a part of your life and where your focus needs to be right now. Ask Him to reveal potential stumbling blocks or temptations, and eliminate them before they become a habit.

6. *Receive grace when you stumble.* Your goal is not perfection but to make changes that result in life-long healthy habits. To accomplish this, you may have to stumble a few times before you can identify areas in which you are weaker than you realize. When you stumble, receive the Lord's grace and ap-ply what you have learned to your plan for change.

7. *Celebrate your successes.* One of the best ways to develop a good habit is to reinforce positive behavior. When you achieve a goal you've been working on, celebrate your victory and reward yourself. Do some-thing that supports your new behavior and doesn't sabotage it: Spend time with a friend, get a massage or watch a good movie.

As you persevere through the change process, you train for the disciplined life the Lord wants you to live, which will produce His righteousness and peace within you.

past failures—and past successes

Forgetting what is behind and straining toward what is ahead,
I press on toward the goal to win the prize for which God has
called me heavenward in Christ Jesus.

PHILIPPIANS 3:13-14

Becoming a new creation in Christ means that we need to put our past failures as well as our successes in the proper perspective. Past failures have the power to paralyze us if we let them. Have you ever found yourself thinking, *I have failed so many times that I just don't have the courage to try again*? Fear of failure because of past experiences can keep us from success in the future.

Not only do past failures have the ability to affect our progress, but so do past successes. Have you ever found yourself thinking, *I lost weight before, but I know I can't be that successful again; I'm older now*. Past successes can place limitations on what God wants to do in our life. Like the apostle Paul, we must adopt the perspective he shared in Philippians 3:13-14: "Brothers [and sisters], I do not consider myself yet to have taken hold of it. But one thing I do: Forgetting what is behind and straining toward what is ahead, I press on toward the goal to win the prize for which God has called me heavenward in Christ Jesus."

Paul outlines three actions for us to emulate: *forget what is behind, focus on what is ahead* and *press on toward the prize.*

FORGET WHAT IS BEHIND

What in Paul's life did he need to forget? Perhaps it was his successes, his education or his religious standing. Of course, even Paul had failures that could weigh him down if he were to dwell on them, such as his intense persecution of Christians before his encounter with Jesus on the road to Damascus (see Acts 9:1-19).

Identify at least one recent failure that has the potential to weigh you down. How has this failure affected your view of the transforming power of God in your life?

_____

_____

_____

_____

_____

God has a purpose for everything. Can you think of a way in which God might use this failure to accomplish His plan in your life? Explain.

_____

_____

_____

_____

_____

Forgetting what is behind does not mean having spiritual amnesia, but it does mean that we do not allow the past to have power over us today.

FOCUS ON WHAT IS AHEAD

Of what could Paul have been thinking when he wrote the words "straining toward what is ahead"? Perhaps he was remembering the words of Jeremiah 29:11: "'For I know the plans I have for you,' declares the LORD, 'plans to prosper you and not to harm you, plans to give you hope and a future.'"

Perhaps Paul had called to mind the words of Isaiah 43:18-19: "Forget the former things; do not dwell on the past. See, I am doing a new thing! Now it springs up; do you not perceive it? I am making a way in the desert and streams in the wasteland." Do you believe that these words of our great God and Savior are true for your life?

Straining toward what is ahead means striving toward our bright new future! God is making a way in the desert for us to be successful.

Identify one new thing you have perceived that God is doing in your life to turn your desert into an oasis.

_____

_____

_____

_____

_____

PRESS ON TOWARD THE PRIZE

Pressing on means that we don't give up, even when our circumstances feel overwhelming. "For the LORD your God is the one who goes with you to fight for you against your enemies to give you victory" (Deuteronomy 20:4). There are days when you will actually feel God pushing you with His strong right arm, helping you to press on.

Identify some things in your life that discourage you from pressing on.

_____

_____

_____

_____

_____

_____

_____

_____

Now spend some time in prayer, asking God to push you past that discouragement and help you keep pressing on, even in your weakest moments. Here are some words to get you started. You may want to record your entire prayer in your prayer journal.

Dear Lord, thank You for Paul's encouragement
to leave my past failures and successes behind, to strain toward
my bright future and to press on—even in the difficult times.
I know that I can accomplish these things in Your strength . . .

Body

LEARN IT

- A healthy weight-loss goal and appropriate calorie range
- The importance of quality food in appropriate quantities
- Physical activity options

LIVE IT

The Live It Plan for Food

- Use the information from the United States Department of Agriculture (USDA) MyPyramid guidelines.
- Practice appropriate food choices and portions at every meal and snack.
- Track your daily choices on the Live It Tracker.

The Live It Plan for Physical Activity

- Create a physical-activity lifestyle that's right for you.
- Use the FITT formula (frequency, intensity, time, type) for cardiovascular activity, strength training, flexibility and balance.
- Walk toward a worthy goal.
- Track your daily choices on the Live It Tracker.

the nutrition and fitness
live it plan!

Welcome to the First Place 4 Health Live It Plan! The first part of this section has several goals for you to accomplish so that healthy eating becomes part of your lifestyle, including (1) setting your healthy weight-loss goal, (2) determining your appropriate caloric intake level, (3) choosing correct food portions and varieties based on the latest scientific information found in the USDA's MyPyramid guidelines, (4) learning the powerful difference between healthy and unhealthy fats and the best choices from other food groups, and (5) becoming an expert at reading food labels so that you can choose the healthiest foods.

The goals of the second part of this section are aimed at your making physical movement part of your lifestyle:

- Creating an individualized exercise program combining cardiovascular, strength-training and flexibility and balance exercises and your preferred lifestyle activities.
- Applying exercise recommendations based on your current physical assessment.
- Making physical movement a daily part of your life, no matter how busy your schedule is.
- Adding years to your life.

These two sections combined—*nutrition* and *fitness*—are called the Live It Plan. Why "Live It"? Because God provides abundant life through Jesus, His Son; when we follow Jesus, not only is abundant life a spiritual reality, but it also is a physical reality and pertains to the choices we make to live according to God's best plan for our optimum physical health. This plan includes the food we eat.

The best food plan is one that doesn't feel like a diet. So take a deep breath and get ready to delete old self-talk and to record over your preconceptions of what it means to make healthy choices about eating *and* exercise!

The Live It Plan encompasses two aspects of your physical health: nutrition and physical activity. Both are essential to weight management.

Overweight and obesity are much more than cosmetic concerns. Approximately 300,000 deaths each year are attributed to obesity. But this is a lifestyle disease that can be avoided by healthy choices. The primary causes of overweight and obesity are (1) increased caloric consumption (too many calories in), and (2) decreased energy output (not enough calories out).

Were you hoping for a different answer? (At least it's a simple one.) When we consume more calories than our body needs, and we fail to burn those excess calories due to an increasingly sedentary lifestyle, we store the unused calories as fat.

However, the good news is twofold:

1 You can break free from the bondage of overweight and obesity by changing the way you eat and the way you move.

2 Even a modest weight loss can improve your health.

The Live It Plan is not another deprivation diet that you won't be able to stick with no matter how hard you try. The Live It Plan teaches you how to bring your weight to a healthy level by *choosing healthy foods in proper portions for your level of lifestyle activity*. That's it.

It's simple, but it's not always easy. But here's more good news: You don't have to figure this out by yourself, and you'll receive lots of encouragement along the way. First Place 4 Health will give you the necessary tools to make the necessary changes, and your First Place 4 Health leader and fellow group members will encourage you and keep you accountable (in a grace-filled way) to walk the road to total health. It's a simple road that requires consistent steps in the same direction.

The road you will walk requires that you take three steps, which will be explained in the following pages:

1 **Learn** that change begins on the inside—investigate why you haven't been able to maintain significant weight loss in the past.

2 **Choose** to readjust your attitude, your environment and your behavior to ready yourself for success.

3 **Use** all the tools First Place 4 Health provides, including group encouragement, to make small, positive changes every day that will eventually lead you to total health.

Let's begin!

Step One

learn that change begins
from the inside out.

You may be thinking, *Just tell me what to do, and I'll do it.* It is completely understandable that you'd like to jump right into the First Place 4 Health eating guidelines. But you need to do something first, or at least you need to do something else while you're learning about food and exercise choices. This first thing—doing a little bit of interior work—will make a positive difference in helping you achieve your health goals. When you understand your motivations in the area of food choices, you can begin to redirect your course onto the right path. In fact, doing this work will make all the difference in achieving your goal of permanent weight loss.

Although it's possible that you don't have any emotional issues surrounding your weight, most people can't achieve permanent, lasting weight loss unless they have investigated the various ways they have used food to fill the empty places that have nothing to do with physical hunger. Taking a look at the way you handle your emotions is not a side trip or a detour. This path leads directly to your destination, and you won't get there without consulting this particular map.

If you haven't yet investigated your history with food and how you have used food to cope with nonphysical issues, reread the Emotions section of this guide and work through that section again while you're learning how to use the MyPyramid nutrition guidelines. You will need to set aside time to work through the section, and you'll need your Bible and a writing journal. If you are tempted to forget about doing this, remember that success is in the total process. Your understanding of the need for change precedes the change. In other words, to change your current behavior regarding food and physical activity, you will need to change the thoughts that created an imbalanced relationship with food and exercise.

MENTAL FOOD FIGHTS

Here's a digest version if you haven't yet turned to the Emotions section of your guide. Reading this won't take the place of doing the needed self-assessment, but see if any of the answers on the following page sound familiar.

Why are you overweight?

"I don't have time to cook and make healthy meals."

"I have to eat out a lot because of my job."

"My kids want the junk food, so I can't help being around it."

Blaming others is unproductive. Being honest with yourself is a first step in the right direction. Maybe you've used food to cope with a stressful job or the loss of a loved one. Or perhaps you developed certain eating habits when you were younger and have continued to practice them even though you're less physically active now. Whatever the reason, it's time to face the truth and let it help you break away from the bondage of using food to cope.

Why do you want to lose weight?

"To look better in my clothes."

"To lower my cholesterol and prevent a heart attack."

"So that I can play with my kids outside for longer than 10 minutes."

The last two reasons will be stronger allies as you make positive changes regarding food intake and physical activity. Looks come and go, but good health will always matter to your family, your friends and yourself! We've learned from fad diets and quick-fix traps that getting thin quickly will not necessarily guarantee happiness or health. Adopting and embracing a healthy lifestyle encourage the maintenance of a healthy weight and fitness level and will bring happiness in addition to health.

If you've lost weight in the past, why did you gain it back?

"The food plan was too strict and complicated."

"I didn't have any support from the people around me."

"It was a really hard year, and I just couldn't stick with it."

These answers sound sort of familiar, don't they? What types of circumstances or thoughts trigger your relapse into unhealthy patterns of behavior? When you figure out what drives you to relapse, you can use that knowledge to prepare and plan for the inevitable bumps in your journey. Knowing the kind of circumstances that trip you up is important to the process of developing a healthy lifestyle.

To complete **Step One,** answer these three questions for yourself:

1 Why are you overweight? _____

2. Why do you want to lose weight? _____

3 If you've lost weight in the past, why did you gain it back? _____

_____

choose to set yourself up
for success!

I f you've been working on uncovering the root issues surrounding your weight gain and your motivations for losing weight, your next step is to plan for success! This involves assessing what types of things influence your behavior the most and how to change what has a negative influence on you.

A vast number of studies show a strong relationship between an individual's environment and behavior. Your *view of self* refers to your attitudes and beliefs. *Environment* comprises both your physical and social settings. *Behavior* is related to weight loss and weight management, which might include practicing portion control, cooking healthy at home and exercising most days of the week. Understanding and anticipating the interaction between these three elements is the basis of how to set yourself up for success.

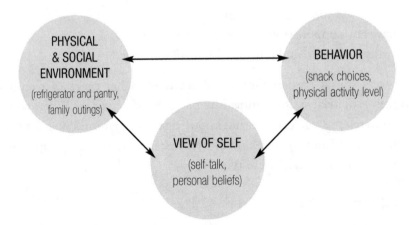

Figure 1. The Dynamic Relationship Between Self, Behavior and Environment. Adapted from Albert Bandura's model of reciprocal determinism. Albert Bandura, *Social Cognitive Theory* (1989), quoted in Ross Vasta, ed., *Six Theories of Child Development* (London: Jessica Kingsley Publishers, 1992), pp. 1-60.

PHYSICAL AND SOCIAL ENVIRONMENT

Both your physical environment and your social environment affect your behavior and your view of self. Let's look at them one at a time.

Physical Environment

Out of sight, out of mind. This saying might not be an absolute truth for you, but when it comes to your food environment, you can benefit from heeding that advice. For example, if you struggle with eating desserts throughout the day or after every meal, one solution would be to simply remove them from your physical environment (out of your refrigerator, pantry, car, closet, desk—wherever they are). The same solution applies to regular soda, fat-laden snacks and processed foods that offer little nutritional value but plenty of calories. Conversely, you can promote healthy eating by making nutritious items available in your physical environment. If you don't have healthy options to choose from, chances are you won't choose them at all.

Social Environment

If your idea of a Friday night with friends or family includes a huge meal at your favorite restaurant, followed by a movie with high-fat, high-sugar treats, it's time for a change! Your social environment is a critical factor in making (or breaking) those healthy habits you're trying to develop. In fact, social support, or the lack of it, is a proven psychological determinant of health behavior change. You need to encourage others and be encouraged by others to make positive changes in your everyday life. Changing your social environment can be difficult—you may meet resistance from people who don't have your same goals, or you may even meet resistance within yourself—but try to do everything possible to make your social calendar fit with your weight-loss and health-improvement agenda.

VIEW OF SELF

Your attitudes, beliefs and self-talk (repetitious thoughts you tell yourself) are another strong influence affecting your behavior and your physical and social settings. For example, how you view yourself with regard to what you deserve or what you are capable of doing alters the path you take, making it either more or less difficult. Perceived self-efficacy (believing that you are capable) is a key ingredient to successful accomplishment of any task. A strong sense of self-efficacy encourages you to reach your goals and gives you a sense of well-being by:

- providing confidence to approach a difficult task as a challenge instead of a threat,
- encouraging strong commitment to the task,
- enabling quick recovery regardless of setbacks, and
- assuring control over threats to accomplishing the task.

If you don't have a strong sense of your capability to reach your goals, you're more likely to:

- shy away from difficult tasks and see them as personal threats,
- have low aspirations and weak commitment to goals,
- dwell on your shortcomings and on the obstacles in your path,
- give up too quickly and fail to recover from setbacks, and
- fall easy victim to stress and depression.

All is not lost if you recognize yourself in the second group of characteristics. First Place 4 Health recognizes that your personal environment—your attitudes and thoughts—is a major influence on your journey to total health. We will provide tools throughout this book to retrain your mind and help you record over any destructive thought tapes that are sabotaging your success (see more in both the Mind and Emotions sections in this guide).

BEHAVIOR

Behaviors that are related to weight loss and weight management range from preparing dinner at home most nights of the week to cutting your food in half at restaurants and packing up half of it to go. Some behaviors will be easier to adopt than others. But all of these suggestions will make your physical and social settings, as well as your personal attitudes and beliefs, conducive to whatever behaviors you need to adopt.

1. Clear Out "Toxic" Foods from Your Immediate Physical Environment

Clean out your refrigerator, your pantry, your desk drawer, your closet, your car—wherever you find the wrong edibles! Don't wait for the food to disappear later in the week—clear out the junk *today*. This includes high-fat, high-calorie and nutritionally empty foods and beverages. Eating some of these in moderation is one thing, but a food environment consisting of "staples o' junk" is quite another.

Send the following foods on a long vacation:

- Regular soft drinks and other sugar-filled beverages
- Fried foods
- Non-whole-grain bread and pasta
- High-calorie sweets
- High-fat dairy products (milk, cheese, yogurt, ice cream and whipped cream)

2. Make a List of Food-Free Activities that You Consider Treats

Think of the many available things that are fun and food-free, and then make a list of these that you can keep handy. You can find great emotional satisfaction away from food.

Treat yourself to constructive activities after periods of regular exercise or other sustained healthy behaviors.

Is it difficult for you to think of nonfood treats? Try these:

- Take a walk outside.
- Write in a journal.
- Visit a neighbor or friend.
- Go to a local art gallery.
- Purchase home-repair supplies at your local DIY store.
- Take your dog to a park.
- Get lost in your favorite bookstore.
- Sit in the sunshine with a good book.
- Get a manicure or a pedicure.
- Plan a vacation or long weekend away from home.
- Review last week's sermon notes while enjoying a hot cup of tea.

3. Get Support

Commit to attend your First Place 4 Health group every week and have at least one supportive person (First Place 4 Health member or not) who knows what you're doing. This could be your spouse, a friend, a neighbor or a coworker. Prayerfully consider who will be your voice of encouragement and accountability.

To complete **Step Two,** do these three things:

1 Clear out "toxic" foods from your immediate physical environment. List some of these below.

_____

_____

2 Make a list of food-free activities that you consider treats:

_____

_____

_____

3 Get support! Write down the name of at least one person you feel could provide support to you on this journey:

_____

_____

_____

use the tools provided in the live it plan !

The First Place 4 Health nutrition plan is uncomplicated, straightforward and good for life! Based on credible science and common sense, it provides 100-percent fad-free, gimmickless advice that will not only help you lose weight but will also pave your way to better health. Most diets really just include the same principles over and over again but with new packaging and a few bogus claims tucked in for marketing purposes. Despite all the hype, the bottom line is still the same: *calories in versus calories out*. However, the calories you take in should be delicious, enjoyable and contribute not only to weight maintenance but also to health enhancement! Remember, this is the LIVE It, not the DIE It!

The only catch is that you have to *do* it.

You already have a good idea of what is healthy and what is not. The bridge that connects knowledge and action is a narrow one. Successful passage requires a purposeful direction, a prayerful heart and acknowledgment of the issues discussed in steps 1 and 2, which are crucial to total health and long-term weight management.

First Place 4 Health is *not* designed to teach you how to continue eating poorly while losing weight. It is a plan that will teach you to choose what is better for your health and your waistline, every day. As defined by the *Dietary Guidelines for Americans 2005*, a healthy diet is one that "emphasizes fruits, vegetables, whole grains, and fat-free or low-fat milk and milk products; includes lean meats, poultry, fish, bean, eggs, and nuts; and is low in saturated fats, trans fats, cholesterol, salt (sodium), and added sugars."[1] That definition guides the First Place 4 Health Live-It recommendations. They are practical, realistic, flexible and delicious.

Note

1. U.S. Department of Health and Human Services and U.S. Department of Agriculture, *Dietary Guidelines for Americans, 2005,* 6th ed. (Washington, DC: U.S. Government Printing Office, January 2005).

the nutrition top 10!

There are 20 principles in the Live It Plan: 10 are about nutrition and 10 are about fitness (we'll get to those in part 2 of this section of the guide). For now, read slowly and thoughtfully through the 10 principles about nutrition. Here you will find timeless rules of conduct to help you achieve healthy, successful weight loss.

1. Set Realistic and Different Goals

Take an honest look at where your weight is now and where you desire it to be. Embrace the reality that your weight-loss journey may last much longer than 12 weeks, and set your goals accordingly. Gradual weight loss (no more than two pounds a week) is secondary to lifestyle change and is the most effective kind of weight loss. Furthermore, there are many other indicators of health besides the number on a scale. Are you physically stronger as the result of increased physical activity? Do you have more energy throughout the day? Have you seen any change in your cholesterol level or blood pressure? Health and wellness are *not* determined just by weight.

2. Plan Ahead and Prioritize

You are the only one who can make the choices that place your health at a high priority. You must be intentional about preparing your home, office, car and calendar to be a safe haven for healthy eating. Achieving your goals can only be accomplished by having a plan that you strongly believe in and then relentlessly acting upon it.

3. Concentrate on Quality

Stop focusing on "good" and "bad" foods by focusing on making healthy food choices. You're not cheating when you eat unhealthy; you're *choosing*. Choose what is better and begin reaping the benefits. For example, allot at least half of your grain choices as whole grains—leave out the white stuff. Fill up on fiber-rich and juicy fruits and vegetables—at least five to seven every day. Go lean with protein by choosing trim meats and poultry as well as fish and beans. Switch to low-fat (skim or 1%) milk and milk products, and be sure you choose enough calcium-rich foods. Select unsaturated oils, and cut out foods high in saturated fat, added sugar and sodium. (See "Focus on Fruits" and the five articles that follow it for healthier choices from each group.)

4. Quantity Counts

Many of us suffer from portion distortion. Eating too much of anything (healthy or unhealthy) can lead to weight gain. Learn what an appropriate portion size is by reading labels, measuring food portions a few times until you can trust your perception and making educated estimates when you must. Get accustomed to cutting your portions in half at most restaurants or splitting them with a friend or family member. Forget supersizing anything! (See "A Cure for Portion Distortion" for details.)

5. Begin with a Healthy Breakfast

Even when you're not hungry, you will want to jumpstart your metabolism for the day with a balanced breakfast eaten up to four hours after waking. People who eat breakfast generally burn 4 to 6 percent more calories than those who don't, and they eat fewer calories throughout the day![1] Not only does eating breakfast help your body function more efficiently, but it also protects you from overeating.

6. Choose Better Beverages

Your beverage choice impacts your weight and your health. Most Americans consider only the calories of solid foods, but did you know that beverages supply nearly a quarter of our total calories? And the largest contributors of these calories are nutrient-poor, sweetened beverages, according to national surveys.[2] Replace such beverages as regular soda, presweetened teas and fruit-flavored drinks with water and water-based, calorie-free beverages, low-fat milk and 100-percent juices with no added sugar.

7. Spread Your Calories Around

Take your estimated calorie range and divide it by three meals and two snacks. The meals/snacks don't have to be equal in calories, but the goal is to eat every three to five hours when awake rather than waiting until your stomach is growling uncontrollably! (You may need to eat something every two to three hours or so if you're dealing with control of blood-sugar levels.) Try to get the majority of your calories in by midafternoon, and end the day with a lighter dinner.

8. Balance Your Plate

To create a nutritionally balanced and complete meal or snack, divide every meal and snack into three components: some *quality* carbohydrate, protein and fat in the appropriate *quan-*

tities (see numbers 3 and 4 of the Nutrition Top 10). A few examples of balanced snacks include fruit, nuts and yogurt; hummus, cheese and crackers; an apple and peanut butter; berries and cottage cheese.

9. Read Food Labels

Become a proactive, health-conscious consumer by reading and comparing food labels, nutrition facts and ingredients lists. Nutrition facts are also provided at most restaurants and even online. Everything you need to know to make an informed decision about anything from applesauce to zucchini bread can be found by simply flipping the item over and reading the entire label. (See "Understanding the Nutrition Facts Panel.")

10. Practice Mindfulness

Using your Live It Tracker, keep a written record of what you eat and drink. This exercise will make you aware of your motivations and choices. Are you truly hungry or are you tired, bored or upset? This exercise will also remind you to eat slowly and savor your meals—you'll enjoy them much better this way. Relearn what hunger really feels like, and listen to your internal hunger cues—stop when you are full. God designed you with thousands of fascinating intricacies, which all have a purpose. Trust your gut—God made that, too!

Notes

1. Meg Jordan, "Fit Not Fat at 40-Plus: The Shape-Up Plan That Balances Your Hormones, Boosts Your Metabolism, and Fights Female Fat in Your Forties—and Beyond," *Prevention*, October 2002), p. 105.
2. *What America Drinks* is a comprehensive analysis of U.S. beverage consumption that was conducted by Environ International Corporation. The report analyzed data from more than 10,000 Americans ages four and older who participated in the government's National Health and Nutrition Examination Survey 1999-2000 and 2001-2002 and provided reasonable dietary reports of food/beverage intakes. Relationships between selected patterns of beverage use, nutrient intakes and body mass index were examined.

your health
assessment!

When beginning any weight-loss program, it's important to know where you are in terms of standard measures of health. We encourage you to make an appointment with your physician to receive a comprehensive evaluation, including checks of blood pressure, blood lipid levels and glucose tolerance, and other diagnostic tests.

Body weight, size and composition all contribute to an accurate and complete assessment. You can find your numbers and begin to set goals by determining some basic numbers now.

WAIST-TO-HIP RATIO AND WAIST SIZE

Where you carry your weight is related to the health risks associated with obesity. People who tend to put on weight around their middle and above have a greater chance of developing heart disease, abnormal cholesterol levels, high blood pressure and diabetes. A popular way to describe this type of fat distribution is apple-shaped. People who carry their extra weight below the waistline or on their hips, for example, don't seem to have as high a risk for developing these conditions. A popular way of describing this type of fat distribution is pear-shaped.

To determine your waist-to-hip ratio (WHR), ask someone to take your measurements, to ensure accuracy. Have them measure around the smallest part of your waist in inches; don't pull your stomach in, just stand relaxed. The narrowest part of your waistline is usually at the level of or near your belly button. Next, have the person measure your hips in inches at the widest part of your buttocks. Then divide your waist measurement by your hip measurement.

WHR = waist (inches) ÷ hip (inches)

A healthy WHR is below 0.8 if you're a woman, or below 0.9 if you're a man. For both men and women, a WHR of 1.0 or higher is considered "at risk" for heart disease and other problems associated with being overweight. Record your waist size, hip size and waist-to-hip ratio below:

My waist size: _____

My hip size: _____

My waist-to-hip ratio: _____

Your waist size alone is also a good measure of health. Your goal for your waist size is less than 35 inches if you're a woman, or less than 40 inches if you're a man.

Pay attention to both your waist-to-hip ratio and your waist size as you begin eating healthier and exercising. *These are often better indicators of health and weight loss than the number on a scale.*

BODY MASS INDEX

Body mass index (BMI) is the ratio of weight to height and is a rough but reliable indicator of body fatness. BMI does not measure body fat directly; but it is an easy and inexpensive alternative for direct measures of body fat (underwater weighing, for example). BMI has become a key parameter in classifying overweight and obesity. Calculate BMI by dividing your weight in pounds by height in inches squared and multiplying by a conversion factor of 703.

Here's an example:

Weight = 150 pounds; height = 5'5"

Multiply 65 inches by 65 to get height squared ($65 \times 65 = 4{,}225$).

Divide weight by height squared ($150 \div 4{,}225 = .0355$).

Multiply that number by 703 ($.0355 \times 703 = 24.95$).

BMI is 24.95.

Now calculate the BMI for your body.

My weight: _____

My height: _____

My BMI: _____

Body Mass Index Table

	Normal						Overweight					Obese										Extreme Obesity															
BMI	19	20	21	22	23	24	25	26	27	28	29	30	31	32	33	34	35	36	37	38	39	40	41	42	43	44	45	46	47	48	49	50	51	52	53	54
Height (inches)												Body Weight (pounds)																								
58	91	96	100	105	110	115	119	124	129	134	138	143	148	153	158	162	167	172	177	181	186	191	196	201	205	210	215	220	224	229	234	239	244	248	253	258
59	94	99	104	109	114	119	124	128	133	138	143	148	153	158	163	168	173	178	183	188	193	198	203	208	212	217	222	227	232	237	242	247	252	257	262	267
60	97	102	107	112	118	123	128	133	138	143	148	153	158	163	168	174	179	184	189	194	199	204	209	215	220	225	230	235	240	245	250	255	261	265	271	276
61	100	106	111	116	122	127	132	137	143	148	153	158	164	169	174	180	185	190	195	201	206	211	217	222	227	232	238	243	248	254	259	264	269	275	280	285
62	104	109	115	120	126	131	136	142	147	153	158	164	169	175	180	186	191	196	202	207	213	218	224	229	235	240	246	251	256	262	267	273	278	284	289	295
63	107	113	118	124	130	135	141	146	152	158	163	169	175	180	186	191	197	203	208	214	220	225	231	237	242	248	254	259	265	270	278	282	287	293	299	304
64	110	116	122	128	134	140	145	151	157	163	169	174	180	186	192	197	204	209	215	221	227	232	238	244	250	256	262	267	273	279	285	291	296	302	308	314
65	114	120	126	132	138	144	150	156	162	168	174	180	186	192	198	204	210	216	222	228	234	240	246	252	258	264	270	276	282	288	294	300	306	312	316	324
66	118	124	130	136	142	148	155	161	167	173	179	186	192	198	204	210	216	223	229	235	241	247	253	260	266	272	278	284	291	297	303	309	315	322	328	334
67	121	127	134	140	146	153	159	166	172	178	185	191	198	204	211	217	223	230	236	242	249	255	261	268	274	280	287	293	299	306	312	319	325	331	338	344
68	125	131	138	144	151	158	164	171	177	184	190	197	203	210	216	223	230	236	243	249	256	262	269	276	282	289	295	302	308	315	322	328	335	341	348	354
69	128	135	142	149	155	162	169	176	182	189	196	203	209	216	223	230	236	243	250	257	263	270	277	284	291	297	304	311	316	324	331	338	345	351	358	365
70	132	139	146	153	160	167	174	181	188	195	202	209	216	222	229	236	243	250	257	264	271	278	285	292	299	306	313	320	327	334	341	348	355	362	369	376
71	136	143	150	157	165	172	179	186	193	200	208	215	222	229	236	243	250	257	265	272	279	286	293	301	308	315	322	329	338	343	351	358	365	372	379	386
72	140	147	154	162	169	177	184	191	199	206	213	221	228	235	242	250	258	265	272	279	287	294	302	309	316	324	331	338	346	353	361	368	375	383	390	397
73	144	151	159	166	174	182	189	197	204	212	219	227	235	242	250	257	265	272	280	288	295	302	310	318	325	333	340	348	355	363	371	378	386	393	401	408
74	148	155	163	171	179	186	194	202	210	218	225	233	241	249	256	264	272	280	287	295	303	311	319	326	334	342	350	358	365	373	381	389	396	404	412	420
75	152	160	168	176	184	192	200	208	216	224	232	240	248	256	264	272	279	287	295	303	311	319	327	335	343	351	359	367	375	383	391	399	407	415	423	431
76	156	164	172	180	189	197	205	213	221	230	238	246	254	263	271	279	287	295	304	312	320	328	336	344	353	361	369	377	385	394	402	410	418	426	435	443

Source: Adapted from *Clinical Guidelines on the Identification, Evaluation and Treatment of Overweight and Obesity in Adults: The Evidence Report*

Interpretation of my BMI: _____

BMI	Weight Status
Below 18.5	Underweight
18.5 - 24.9	Normal
25.0 - 29.9	Overweight
30.0 - 39.9	Obese
40.0 and above	Extreme Obesity

BODY WEIGHT

Despite social norms that emphasize body weight above everything else, the quality of your health is determined by much more. Weight should *not* be considered the best and most accurate picture of total health. It is quite possible to be thin and unhealthy at the same time.

Many of us focus way too much on the number shown on our scale. Every body is built differently. Did you know that muscle weighs more than fat? An ideal body weight is specific to each individual and should be considered in conjunction with other measurements.

Make sure you have an accurate measure by using a reliable scale and weighing in the morning after you've voided.

My current weight: _____

Your desired body weight should be a healthy weight you were able to maintain for at least one year after your twenty-first birthday. Be honest and realistic with yourself, and remember that this number is not the most important element in total health. Consider your body type and genetics when determining your desired body weight.

My desired body weight: _____

Your ideal body-weight range is based on weight ranges associated with good health and is determined by two methods that consider your gender, height and frame size: (1) the Metropolitan Height-Weight Tables, and (2) the Hamwi Formula. Both methods provide only rough estimates of ideal body weight, so consider taking an average of the two. Most women have small to medium frames, and most men have medium to large frames. Since everyone is built a little differently, consider a weight *range* as opposed to a single number.

Find the weight range for your height and frame size listed in the appropriate Metropolitan Height-Weight Tables. Note that *the table is not perfect.* Use its range to estimate a weight that seems most realistic for you. During your weight-loss journey, you will find the weight that feels best for you.

METROPOLITAN HEIGHT-WEIGHT TABLES[1]

| WOMEN | | | | MEN | | | |
| Height | Ideal Body Weight Per Frame Size | | | Height | Ideal Body Weight Per Frame Size | | |
Feet/Inches	Small	Medium	Large	Feet/Inches	Small	Medium	Large
4'9"	102-111	109-121	118-131	5'1"	128-134	131-141	138-150
4'10"	103-113	111-123	120-134	5'2"	130-136	133-143	140-153
4'11"	104-115	113-126	122-137	5'3"	132-138	135-145	142-156
5'0"	106-118	115-129	125-140	5'4"	134-140	137-148	144-160
5'1"	108-121	118-132	128-143	5'5"	136-142	139-151	146-164
5'2"	111-124	121-135	131-147	5'6"	138-145	142-154	149-168
5'3"	114-127	124-138	134-151	5'7"	140-148	145-157	152-172
5'4"	117-130	127-141	137-155	5'8"	142-151	148-160	155-176
5'5"	120-133	130-144	140-159	5'9"	144-154	151-163	158-180
5'6"	123-136	133-147	143-163	5'10"	146-157	154-166	161-184
5'7"	126-139	136-150	146-167	5'11"	149-160	157-170	164-188
5'8"	129-142	139-153	149-170	6'0"	152-164	160-174	168-192
5'9"	132-145	142-156	152-173	6'1"	155-168	164-178	172-197
5'10"	135-148	145-159	155-176	6'2"	158-172	167-182	176-202
5'11"	138-151	148-162	158-179	6'3"	162-176	171-187	181-207

THE HAMWI FORMULA[2]

For men, consider 106 pounds for your first five feet in height. Add six pounds for every inch thereafter. Add and subtract 10 percent of this number to create a weight range.

For women, consider 100 pounds for your first five feet in height. Add five pounds for every inch thereafter. Add and subtract 10 percent of this number to create a weight range.

Here's an example:

A male 5'10" tall
Consider 106 pounds for the first 5 feet in height.
Multiply 10×6 ($10 \times 6 = 60$).
Add 60 to 106 ($60 + 106 = 166$).
Take 10% of 166 ($166 \times 0.10 = 16.6$).
Determine ± 10% weight range ($166 - 16.6$) to ($166 + 16.6$).
His ideal body-weight range is 149 to 183 (rounded to the nearest pound).

My ideal body-weight range: _____

THE SECRETS OF SUCCESSFUL WEIGHT LOSS[3]

Haven't you always wanted to know how people who lose weight keep it off? Here are some of the behavioral characteristics of the members of the National Weight Control Registry, an ongoing project that tracks people who successfully lose weight and keep if off. The Live It Plan for nutrition and physical activity incorporates many of these tips for success!

They learned portion sizes and practice control.

They keep a diary of their eating.

They exercise consistently.

They changed their attitude and self-talk to be more constructive.

They have a coach or other source of social support.

They changed their environment to be conducive to health and their goals.

They plan ahead of time, stay organized and anticipate triggers that could get them off track.

They made a healthy lifestyle their everyday lifestyle.

They focus on their health, not just their appearance.

They eat breakfast daily.

They eat lower-fat meals and snacks.

They weigh themselves once a week or measure themselves every month to monitor progress.

Now it's time to set a healthy weight-loss goal for the current 12-week session. Remember to set a goal that is a realistic and personalized. Even a modest weight loss can result in significant health benefits.[4] Multiply your current weight by 0.9 to determine what a weight loss of 10 percent would be for you. Divide this number by five pounds to determine how many months it will take you to reach your goal if you lose one to two pounds per week (a safe and effective rate of weight loss). Setting long-range goals is important, but try to focus on your short-term weight loss goal *first*—that is, your weight loss goal for the next 12 weeks. This is especially important if you have a lot of weight to lose. Take it day by day and session by session, and remember that gradual weight loss is safest and most effective.

Lose
28.71 lbs
5 months

Notes

1. Adapted from the Metropolitan Life Insurance Company, estimates include weight of indoor clothing (5 pounds for men, 3 pounds for women).
2. G. J. Hamwi, "Therapy: Changing Dietary Concepts," in *Diabetes Mellitus: Diagnosis and Treatment*, vol. 1, ed. T. S. Danowski (New York: American Diabetes Association, 1964), pp. 73-78.
3. The dietary recommendations of the First Place 4 Health program are based on the most recent Dietary Guidelines for Americans and the MyPyramid system published by the United States Department of Agriculture and Department of Health and Human Services. Both agencies provide science-based guidelines on the most current and relevant medical and scientific knowledge available. In addition to reliance on these federal resources, the Live It Plan recommendations have been shaped by advice provided by participants in the National Weight Control Registry. The National Weight Registry, established in 1994 by Drs. Rena Wing and James O. Hill, was developed to identify and investigate the characteristics of individuals who have succeeded at maintaining their weight loss of 30 pounds or more for at least one year. The registry currently tracks more than 5,000 individuals who fall into that esteemed category. Detailed questionnaires and annual surveys are used to examine the behavioral and psychological characteristics of those who maintain significant weight loss, as well as the strategies they use to maintain their weight loss.
4. G. Oster and others, "Lifetime Health and Economic Benefits of Weight Loss Among Obese Persons," *American Journal of Public Health*, vol. 89 (October 1999), pp. 1536-1542.

nutrition for life!

A re you familiar with the phrase "Don't work harder, work smarter"? Well, there's a smarter way to lose weight than what you may be used to. Although you can lose weight from a number of different diets, how much of that weight loss can you maintain after one month, six months or a year? Adopting a healthy lifestyle over the length of your life will not only help you lose those unwanted pounds but will also give you a deeper sense of gratitude for your body (your temple) and for your Creator.

The First Place 4 Health nutrition plan is simple, practical, realistic, flexible and good for life. Even so, it is important that as a First Place 4 Health participant, you *consult a medical or health-care professional before beginning this or any other weight-loss or physical-fitness program.*

In the next several pages, you will find out how to (1) estimate your calorie needs for weight loss, (2) estimate approximately how many servings you need daily of each food group, and (3) eat a variety of foods in moderation.

CHOOSING A CALORIE RANGE

Calories are the energy in the foods and beverages you consume. They provide the fuel that powers your body physically, mentally, emotionally and spiritually. Along with the vast number of nutrients contained in healthy foods and beverages, calories are essential in obtaining adequate nutrition. Furthermore, the key to achieving and maintaining a healthy weight lies in calorie balance.

Weight gain occurs when you take in more calories than your body needs. Similarly, to lose weight you must reduce the number of calories you take in (by adjusting your dietary intake) or increase the number of calories you use up (by increasing your level of physical activity). One pound is equal to 3,500 calories. In order to lose a pound a week, you must reduce your daily intake by 500 calories, increase your physical activity to burn 500 calories a day, or balance the deficit between both dietary intake and physical expenditure.

There are various methods for estimating an individual's calorie needs. Personal variables such as height, weight, age, sex, activity level and other factors all play a role in tailoring the estimation. It is important to remember that most methods provide only an estimate, not an exact determination, of calorie needs.

It's best to lose weight slowly, at a rate of one to two pounds per week; so if you feel that your calorie range is a little too low, for example, feel free to tailor it by adding 100 to 200 calories and vice versa. Low-calorie diets and rapid weight loss promote a slowing of the metabolic rate, which makes it more difficult to lose and maintain your weight in the long run. Also, on such diets you often lose more lean body mass and water than fat. Your goal should be fat loss, not loss of water or muscle.

If you have a very large amount of weight to lose (100 pounds or more) and feel that the following calorie ranges are too restrictive, consider the following:

- When determining a realistic calorie range for weight loss, it is important to know how much you are actually eating to begin with. Determine this first by using your Live It Tracker to trace how many calories you typically consume in an average day. Track your intake for three days and then take an average. The point of this exercise is to determine your typical (pre-First Place 4 Health) intake so as to better gauge what an appropriate and realistic deficit of calories would be to promote *gradual* fat loss. Be honest, and do not adjust your intake for this exercise.

- Next, based on your typical caloric intake, determine what a challenging but realistic reduction in calories would be for you. A deficit of even 300 to 500 calories per day will prevent further gain and lead to gradual weight loss for most people. For example, if someone typically consumes 2,500 calories per day, a reduction of 500 calories to yield 2,000 daily calories will make a difference. The bottom line is that, based on your current weight, you may need to add 200 to 300 calories to what is listed in the chart below; and that is perfectly fine. We simply ask that you commit to reassessing your needs once you begin to lose, and consider gradually tapering your calorie range to the suggested range.

- Much of this process of determining an appropriate calorie range involves trial and error, so begin with a calorie range you can live with and reassess every few weeks. Focus on making healthy behavior changes (like eating more fruits and vegetables and less fat-laden meals and snacks), and trust that the numbers will work themselves out eventually. The last thing we want you to do is try a calorie range that is too low, get frustrated and give up! We also do not want you to consistently lose more than two pounds per week, because it is physiologically impossible to lose more than two pounds of *fat* in that short a time!

Recommended Calorie Ranges for Weight Loss for Adult Women[1]

AGE	ACTIVITY LEVEL 1* (CALORIES PER DAY)	ACTIVITY LEVEL 2** (CALORIES PER DAY)	ACTIVITY LEVEL 3*** (CALORIES PER DAY)
19-20	1700-1800	1900-2000	2100-2200
21-25	1700-1800	1900-2000	2100-2200
26-30	1500-1600	1700-1800	2100-2200
31-35	1500-1600	1700-1800	1900-2000
36-40	1500-1600	1700-1800	1900-2000
41-45	1500-1600	1700-1800	1900-2000
46-50	1500-1600	1700-1800	1900-2000
51-55	1300-1400	1500-1600	1900-2000
56-60	1300-1400	1500-1600	1900-2000
61-65	1300-1400	1500-1600	1700-1800
66-70	1300-1400	1500-1600	1700-1800
71-75	1300-1400	1500-1600	1700-1800
76+	1300-1400	1500-1600	1700-1800

Recommended Calorie Ranges for Weight Loss for Adult Men[2]

AGE	ACTIVITY LEVEL 1* (CALORIES PER DAY)	ACTIVITY LEVEL 2** (CALORIES PER DAY)	ACTIVITY LEVEL 3*** (CALORIES PER DAY)
19-20	2200-2400	2400-2600	2600-2800
21-25	2000-2200	2400-2600	2600-2800
26-30	2000-2200	2200-2400	2600-2800
31-35	2000-2200	2200-2400	2600-2800
36-40	2000-2200	2200-2400	2400-2600
41-45	1800-2000	2200-2400	2400-2600
46-50	1800-2000	2000-2200	2400-2600
51-55	1800-2000	2000-2200	2400-2600
56-60	1800-2000	2000-2200	2200-2400
61-65	1600-1800	2000-2200	2200-2400
66-70	1600-1800	1800-2000	2200-2400
71-75	1600-1800	1800-2000	2200-2400
76+	1600-1800	1800-2000	2000-2200

* Activity Level 1 = 1 to 30 minutes of moderate physical activity a day in addition to daily activities.
** Activity Level 2 = 30 to 60 minutes of moderate physical activity a day in addition to daily activities.
*** Activity Level 3 = More than 60 minutes of moderate physical activity a day in addition to daily activities.
If you'd like to maintain your weight, add 200 calories to both ends of your range.

ALL ABOUT MyPYRAMID

The First Place 4 Health nutrition plan is based on the *USDA MyPyramid Food Guidelines* as well as the most recent *Dietary Guidelines for Americans*. The USDA has been providing food guidance materials to the public since the early twentieth century. MyPyramid, released in April 2005, was revised (1) to reflect the latest nutritional science, including new nutrient standards (such as the dietary reference intakes) and dietary guidelines (published in part by the Department of Health and Human Services); and (2) to help consumers more effectively apply the guidelines through the new graphics, new slogan and an interactive website (www.mypyramid.gov). The MyPyramid symbol encompasses six overarching themes: physical activity, moderation, personalization, proportionality, variety and gradual improvement.

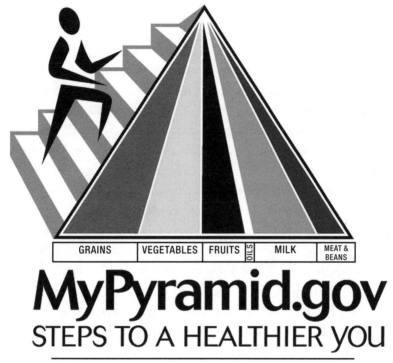

(Image courtesy of the U.S. Department of Agriculture.
The USDA does not endorse any products, services or organizations.)

Physical activity is represented by the person climbing stairs. Daily physical activity is essential not only for weight loss and weight management but also for the prevention of chronic disease and for the enhancement of health.

Moderation in each food group is represented by a narrowing vertical band. The wide base of the band represents foods that should be selected most often, because they have little or no solid fats and/or added sugars. The narrow top represents foods that should be consumed less often, because they contain more solid fats and/or added sugars.

Personalization is the "My" in "MyPyramid." It reminds us that every person is different, and no one specific food plan is right for everybody. At First Place 4 Health you will find the kinds and amounts of food to eat according to your calorie range and based on your personal preferences and tastes.

Proportionality is illustrated by the different widths of the food-group bands, which suggest how much food a person should choose from each group. This, of course, is a general guide. In the following pages you will discover what is right for you.

Variety is symbolized by the six different bands that make up the pyramid, representing the five food groups and oils. Foods from each group provide different nutrients that are all needed for a healthy diet.

Gradual improvement is implied by the slogan for the MyPyramid educational campaign: "Steps to a Healthier You." The slogan encourages gradual improvement as each step in the right direction works to improve diet, physical activity and physical health.

RECOMMENDED FOOD INTAKE BASED ON CALORIE RANGE

The USDA food guide provides suggested amounts of food to consume from the five basic food groups and from oils, to achieve adequate nutrition at several calorie ranges. Nutrient-dense foods (those that provide substantial amounts of nutrients with relatively fewer calories) are represented at the base, the largest portion of the pyramid. These foods are your healthiest options. Such foods include lean meats and fat-free or low-fat milk. However, it is assumed that foods higher in fat and sugar will be consumed occasionally, so they are included in the calculation for daily calories.

Refer to your estimated daily calorie needs to determine which food intake pattern best suits you. Calorie ranges are used because you likely fall in between two levels. Balance your goals between the two and don't worry about being exact. In addition, refer to the Nutrition Top 10 for the basic behavioral changes you need to make. We cannot emphasize enough that your food plan is just *one* aspect of the Live It Plan. (*Note:* This food guide is not to be taken too literally. It is for the purposes of giving you direction on how to disperse your daily calories across the food groups in order to achieve variety, and encouraging a healthy eating lifestyle in order to help you achieve optimum nutrition.)

Beginning with "Focus on Fruits" and ending with "Choosing Healthy Oils," this guide discusses in detail each basic food group and oils; and at the beginning of each article is a table listing foods that we encourage you to: (1) choose *often*, (2) choose *occasionally*, and (3) choose *seldom*.

"Often" foods are the lowest in fat and sugar, and are relatively low in calories. They are also the most nutrient dense. "Occasional" foods are those foods that should be enjoyed every now and then as they do offer nutrition, but at a higher caloric price tag. "Seldom" foods should be enjoyed rarely as they are high-calorie foods with little nutritional value.

Every food can have a place in a healthy diet, but not all foods should have a *prominent* place. As you begin the plan, we encourage you to take a vacation from calorie-dense foods to help jumpstart your weight loss as well as introduce you to a healthier lifestyle of eating.

As your weight loss progresses and you maintain your new weight, you may be able to add some of those foods back into your diet in limited quantities.

Recommended Daily Amount of Food from Each Group[3]

GROUP	DAILY CALORIES							
	1300-1400	1500-1600	1700-1800	1900-2000	2100-2200	2300-2400	2500-2600	2700-2800
Fruits[1]	1.5-2 c.	1.5-2 c.	1.5-2 c.	2-2.5 c.	2-2.5 c.	2.5-3.5 c.	3.5-4.5 c.	3.5-4.5 c.
Vegetables[2]	1.5-2 c.	2-2.5 c.	2.5-3 c.	2.5-3 c.	3-3.5 c.	3.5-4.5 c.	4.5-5 c.	4.5-5 c.
Grains[3]	5 oz-eq.	5-6 oz-eq.	6-7 oz-eq.	6-7 oz-eq.	7-8 oz-eq.	8-9 oz-eq.	9-10 oz-eq.	10-11 oz-eq.
Milk[4]	2-3 c.	3 c.	3 c.	3 c.	3 c.	3 c.	3 c.	3 c.
Meat & Beans[5]	4 oz-eq.	5 oz-eq.	5-5.5 oz-eq.	5.5-6.5 oz-eq.	6.5-7 oz-eq.	7-7.5 oz-eq.	7-7.5 oz-eq.	7.5-8 oz-eq.
Healthy Oils[6]	4 tsp.	5 tsp.	5 tsp.	6 tsp.	6 tsp.	7 tsp.	8 tsp.	8 tsp.

oz-eq. = ounce equivalent, c. = cup, tsp. = teaspoon

1. The fruit group includes all fresh, frozen, canned and dried fruits and fruit juices. In general, 1 cup of fruit, 1 cup of 100-percent fruit juice or $1/2$ cup of dried fruit can be considered 1 cup from the fruit group.

2. The vegetable group includes all fresh, frozen, canned and dried vegetables and vegetable juices. In general, 1 cup of raw or cooked vegetables or vegetable juice, or 2 cups of raw leafy greens can be considered 1 cup from the vegetable group.

3. The grains group includes all foods made from wheat, rice, oats, cornmeal or barley, such as bread, pasta, oatmeal, breakfast cereals, tortillas and grits. In general, 1 slice of bread, 1 cup of ready-to-eat cereal or $1/2$ cup of cooked rice, pasta or cooked cereal can be considered as 1 ounce equivalent from the grains group. Your goal concerning this group is to make at least half of your choices whole grain.

4. The milk group includes all fluid milk, milk products, and foods made from milk that retain their calcium content, such as yogurt and cheese. Foods made from milk that have little to no calcium—such as cream cheese, cream and butter—are not part of the group. Most milk-group choices should be fat-free or low-fat. In general, 1 cup of milk or yogurt, 1-$1/2$ ounces of natural cheese, and 2 ounces of processed cheese can be considered 1 cup from the milk group.

5. One ounce of lean meat, poultry or fish; 1 egg; 1 tablespoon peanut butter; $1/4$ cup cooked dry beans; or $1/2$ ounce of nuts and seeds can be considered as 1 ounce equivalent from the meat and beans group.

6. Healthy oils are made from many different plants and from fish and are liquid at room temperature (unsaturated). Examples include canola, corn, olive, soybean and sunflower oils. Some foods are naturally high in oils, like nuts, olives, some fish, and avocados. Foods that are mainly oil include mayonnaise, certain salad dressings, and soft margarine.

Notes

1. Institute of Medicine of the National Academies, *Dietary Reference Intakes for Energy, Carbohydrate, Fiber, Fat, Fatty Acids, Cholesterol, Protein, and Amino Acids* (The National Academies Press, Washington, DC, 2002). Calorie ranges have been adapted by First Place 4 Health to promote weight loss at a safe rate.
2. Ibid.
3. The USDA *Food Intake Patterns* have been adapted by First Place 4 Health to better reflect our recommendations.

using your
live it tracker!

The Live It Tracker is a tool by which you can keep a record of your nutrition and physical activities as well as your spiritual disciplines. If you use it consistently, research has shown that you will find success faster! Completing your Live It Tracker involves the following steps:

1 Write your name, the date, week number, recommended calorie range (as determined in the "Nutrition for Life" section of this book) and your current activity level (circle one of the choices provided).

2 Write two goals for yourself each week, one of which pertains to your food choices and the other to your activity. For example, a food goal might be to "eat three servings of fruit each day" or "limit desserts to two nights this week." An activity goal might be to "take the stairs every day at work."

3 Write the Scripture memory verse for each week on the lines provided. This will serve as a reminder for you to work on memorizing the verse throughout the week.

4 Find your recommended calorie range in the Recommended Daily Amount of Food from Each Group table and note how much food from each food group you should eat each day. Write these values in the blank table on the row that says "Goal Amount."

5 List your food choices on the lines provided for all meals and snacks every day. At the end of each day, estimate your total for each group and write these values on the row that says "Estimate Your Total."

6 Assess your food quantity by using up and down arrows. Indicate if you need to eat more or less of each food group on the row that says "Increase or Decrease?" Just draw a dash if you met your goal and do not need to increase or decrease the number of servings.

7 Provide a description for your spiritual activities (reading your Bible, practicing your Scripture memory verse) and your physical activities (walking 3 miles or lifting weights for 20 minutes). Be sure to include the number of steps, miles or minutes for your physical activities.

8 At the end of each week, assess how you did in achieving your personal goals and basic goals of First Place 4 Health, such as eating high-quality foods in appropriate quantities. Rate your week as "Great," "So-so" or "Not so great."

Live It Tracker

Name: **Sally Smith** My week at a glance: ☒ Great ❑ So-so ❑ Not so great

Date: **8-10-08** Week #: **2** Calorie Range: **1500-1600** My food goal for next week: **choose more whole-grain foods**

Activity Level: None, < 30 min/day, (30-60 min/day), 60+ min/day My activity goal for next week: **walk at least 10,000 steps each day**

Scripture Memory Verse: **"Therefore, if anyone is in Christ, he is a new creation; the old has gone, the**

new has come!" (2 Corinthians 5:17)

RECOMMENDED DAILY AMOUNT OF FOOD FROM EACH GROUP

Group	Daily Calories							
	1300-1400	1500-1600	1700-1800	1900-2000	2100-2200	2300-2400	2500-2600	2700-2800
Fruits	1.5-2 c.	1.5-2 c.	1.5-2 c.	2-2.5 c.	2- 2.5 c.	2.5- 3.5 c.	3.5- 4.5 c.	3.5- 4.5 c.
Vegetables	1.5-2 c.	2-2.5 c.	2.5-3 c.	2.5-3 c.	3- 3.5 c.	3.5- 4.5 c.	4.5- 5 c.	4.5- 5 c.
Grains	5 oz-eq.	5-6 oz-eq.	6-7 oz-eq.	6-7 oz-eq.	7- 8 oz-eq.	8-9 oz-eq.	9-10 oz-eq.	10-11 oz-eq.
Milk	2- 3 c.	3 c.	3 c.	3 c.	3 c.	3 c.	3 c.	3 c.
Meat & Beans	4 oz-eq.	5 oz-eq.	5- 5.5 oz-eq.	5.5- 6.5 oz-eq.	6.5- 7 oz-eq.	7 -7.5 oz-eq.	7- 7.5 oz-eq.	7.5- 8 oz-eq.
Healthy Oils	4 tsp.	5 tsp.	5 tsp.	6 tsp.	6 tsp.	7 tsp.	8 tsp.	8 tsp.

FOOD CHOICES

Breakfast: 1 c whole-grain cereal with 1/2 c 1% milk & 1/2 c berries Lunch: 2 oz. turkey on whole-wheat bread w/ 1 T. light mayo, lettuce, 1/2 large tomato, string cheese, apple

Dinner: 1 c wholewheat pasta, 1/2 c spaghetti sauce, 1 c grilled veggies, 1 c sugar-free pudding Snacks: 8 oz. light yogurt, 1 oz. walnuts, 1/4 c black bean salsa with 1 oz. baked chips

Group	Fruits	Vegetables	Grains	Meat & Beans	Milk	Oils
Goal Amount	1.5-2 c.	2-2.5 c.	5-6 oz.-eq.	3 c.	5 oz.-eq	5 tsp.
Estimate Your Total	1.5 c.	2 c.	6 oz.-eq.	3 c.	5 oz.-eq	5 tsp.
Increase ⬆ or Decrease ⬇ ?	↑	↑	—	—	—	—

PHYSICAL ACTIVITY SPIRITUAL ACTIVITY

Description: kept my pedometer on today, tried a new strength training class Description: FP4H Bible Study, prayer journaling

Steps/Miles/Minutes: 10,321 steps today, strength training class was 1 hr.

FOOD CHOICES

Breakfast: ___ Lunch: ___

Dinner: ___ Snacks: ___

Group	Fruits	Vegetables	Grains	Meat & Beans	Milk	Oils
Goal Amount						
Estimate Your Total						
Increase ⬆ or Decrease ⬇ ?						

PHYSICAL ACTIVITY SPIRITUAL ACTIVITY

Description: ___ Description: ___

Steps/Miles/Minutes: ___

FOOD CHOICES

Breakfast: ___ Lunch: ___

Dinner: ___ Snacks: ___

Group	Fruits	Vegetables	Grains	Meat & Beans	Milk	Oils
Goal Amount						
Estimate Your Total						
Increase ⬆ or Decrease ⬇ ?						

PHYSICAL ACTIVITY SPIRITUAL ACTIVITY

Description: ___ Description: ___

Steps/Miles/Minutes: ___

focus
on fruits!

Choose Often	Choose Occasionally	Choose Seldom
Fresh and frozen fruits, canned fruits packed in water or juice	Dried fruits, fruits canned in light syrup, 100% fruit juice, olives, avocados	Fruits canned in heavy syrup, fruits prepared in butter or cream sauce, coconut

Fruits are nature-made desserts that are also extremely rich in disease-fighting components like antioxidants, fiber and a vast array of vitamins. Most fruits are naturally low in fat, sodium and calories. None have cholesterol. In general, most adults who exercise less than 30 minutes a day in addition to daily activities need at least 1-1/2 to 2 cups of fruit per day. Refer to your calorie range to determine what amount is right for you.

WHAT'S INCLUDED?

Any fruit or 100-percent fruit juice counts as a part of your fruit servings for the day. Choose either fresh, frozen, canned (in juice or water, not syrup) or dried. You can eat them whole, cut up, pureed—however you prefer. The important thing is that you choose a variety of fruits that differ in nutrient content. For the best nutritional value and benefits of dietary fiber, make most of your choices whole or cut-up fruit rather than juice.

WHAT COUNTS AS 1 CUP?

- 1 cup of chopped, sliced, diced, crushed and drained fresh, frozen or canned fruit
- 1 cup of 100-percent juice
- 1/2 cup of dried fruit (1/4 cup dried counts as a half-cup serving of fruit)

126

The following table lists a variety of fruits and how much of each equals 1 cup and a $1/2$ cup. See how easy it is to get your fruit for the day?

FRUIT	AMOUNT THAT COUNTS AS 1 CUP	AMOUNT THAT COUNTS AS $1/2$ CUP
Apple	1 small (~2.5" diameter), $1/2$ large (~3.25" diameter)	$1/2$ small
Applesauce	1 cup	1 snack container (4 oz.)
Banana	1 large (8" to 9" long)	1 small (less than 6" long)
Cantaloupe	1 cup diced or melon balls	1 medium wedge ($1/8$ of a medium melon)
Grapes, seedless	32 count	16 count
Grapefruit	1 medium (~4" diameter)	$1/2$ medium
Mixed Fruit/Fruit Cocktail	1 cup	1 snack container (4 oz.)
Orange	1 large (~3" diameter)	1 small (~2" diameter)
Peach	1 large (~3" diameter), 2 halves canned	1 small (~2" diameter), 1 snack container (4 oz.)
Pear	1 medium	1 snack container (4 oz.)
Pineapple	1 cup chunks, sliced, crushed, raw, cooked or canned, drained	1 snack container (4 oz.)
Plum	3 medium or 2 large	1 large
Raisins	$1/2$ cup	$1/4$ cup
Strawberries	8 large berries	4 large berries
Watermelon	1 small wedge (1" thick)	6 melon balls

Cups of fruit I need a day: _____

HEALTH BENEFITS FROM EATING FRUIT[1]

Many fruits are key sources of potassium, dietary fiber, vitamin C and folic acid—all of which contribute to the prevention of disease and the enhancement of health.

- **Potassium** helps to maintain healthy blood pressure.

- **Dietary fiber** helps reduce blood cholesterol levels and is essential for a happy bowel (less constipation). The high fiber and water content of fruits also helps you feel full longer with fewer calories.

- **Vitamin C** is important for the growth and repair of tissues. It helps heal wounds faster and keeps your gums and teeth healthy.

- **Folic acid** helps the body form new red blood cells. It is especially important for women who are in their first trimester of pregnancy and those of childbearing age who may become pregnant to consume adequate folic acid to prevent neural tube defects, spina bifida and, anencephaly during their baby's development in the womb.

STRATEGIES FOR EATING MORE FRUITS

- Utilize the crisper or fruit drawer of your refrigerator, and stock it well. Keep fruits where you can see them and be reminded to eat them, such as in a bowl on your kitchen table or counter.

- Buy fresh fruits in season when they may be less expensive and at their peak flavor.

- Keep some dried and canned fruits (packed in water or juice, not in syrup) in your pantry.

- Consider convenience when buying fruits—packages of precut fruits provide healthy snacks in seconds.

- Add fruits to salads, breakfast cereals or yogurt.

- Eat fruits for dessert, such as baked apples.

- Buy some convenient individual containers to pack fruits as snacks.

- Grill fruits or add them to kebobs.

- Add dried fruits or fruit chutney to your chicken dishes.

- Freeze 100-percent juice into juice-bar molds for a healthy summer snack.

- Dip fruit in low-fat yogurt or sugar-free pudding.

- Substitute applesauce for oil when baking cakes—it's delicious!

- Create your own fruit and yogurt parfait without all the sugary syrup.

- Mix acidic fruits like oranges, grapefruits, lemons or pineapple with apples, bananas and pears to prevent them from turning brown. You can also pour a little orange juice over them to stop the browning process.

vary your
vegetables

Choose Often	Choose Occasionally	Choose Seldom
Fresh or frozen vegetables without added fat (butter or gravy)	Canned vegetables without salt	Canned vegetables with salt, vegetables prepared in butter or cream sauce, fried vegetables

We all know that vegetables are good for us, but many of us continue to skip them. Perhaps that's because we have a very limited view of what actually counts as a vegetable. With the beautiful assortment of vegetables available to us, and so many methods for cooking them, it is much easier to achieve their daily recommended intake than many people think. Like fruits, vegetables are rich in fiber and packed with nutrients in addition to being low in fat and calories and cholesterol-free. In general, adults who exercise less than 30 minutes a day in addition to daily activities need 2 to 3 cups of vegetables per day.

WHAT'S INCLUDED?

Any vegetable or 100-percent vegetable juice counts as a member of the vegetable group. Vegetables may be raw or cooked; fresh, frozen, canned or dried/dehydrated; whole, cut-up or mashed. When buying canned vegetables, choose ones with no added salt. (*Note:* Dry beans and peas are considered part of both the vegetable and the meat and beans group, so you can be flexible with how you assign them.) Not only do different vegetables provide different nutrients, but they also provide different textures and flavors. Vary your veggies, and keep things interesting by choosing from each subgroup throughout the week.

Here are some examples of vegetables in each of the five vegetable subgroups, from all of which you should eat each week. It would *not* be nutritionally savvy, for example, to eat from only the starchy subgroup. That would be doing your body and taste buds a disservice.

- **Dark Green:** bok choy, broccoli, collard greens, kale, mesclun (a salad mix of assorted small, young, salad leaves), mustard greens, romaine lettuce, spinach, turnip greens, watercress

- **Orange:** acorn squash, butternut squash, carrots, Hubbard squash, pumpkin, sweet potatoes

- **Dry Beans and Peas, or Legumes:** black beans, black-eyed peas, garbanzo beans (chickpeas), kidney beans, lentils, lima beans (mature), navy beans, pinto beans, soy beans, split peas, tofu (bean curd made from soybeans), white beans

- **Starchy:** corn, green peas, lima beans (green), white potatoes

- **Other:** artichokes, asparagus, bean sprouts, beets, Brussels sprouts, cabbage, cauliflower, celery, cucumbers, eggplant, green beans, green or red peppers, iceberg lettuce, mushrooms, okra, onions, parsnips, tomato juice, tomatoes, turnips, wax beans, summer squash or zucchini

HEALTH BENEFITS FROM EATING VEGETABLES

Vegetables provide nutrients that are essential for health and maintenance of your body. When part of an overall healthy diet, they may help reduce the risk of many chronic diseases and other maladies such as stroke and cardiovascular diseases, type-2 diabetes, certain cancers, coronary heart disease, kidney stones, bone loss, gum disease, obesity, high blood pressure, and poor eye and skin health.

Vegetables are prime sources of vitamins A, C and E; potassium; dietary fiber and folic acid—all of which contribute to the prevention of disease and the enhancement of health.

- **Vitamin A** keeps eyes and skin healthy and prevents infections.

- **Vitamin C** is important for the growth and repair of tissues. It helps heal wounds faster and keeps your gums and teeth healthy.

- **Vitamin E** is a powerful antioxidant that protects against cell oxidation.

- **Potassium** helps to maintain a healthy range of blood pressure.

- **Dietary fiber** helps reduce blood cholesterol levels and is essential for a happy bowel (less constipation). The high fiber and water content of vegetables also helps you feel full longer with fewer calories.

- **Folic acid** helps the body form new red blood cells. It is especially important for women in their first trimester of pregnancy and those of childbearing age who may become pregnant to consume adequate folic acid to prevent neural tube defects, spina bifida and anencephaly during their baby's development in the womb.

WHAT COUNTS AS 1 CUP?

- 1 cup of raw or cooked vegetables
- 1 cup of 100-percent vegetable juice
- 2 cups of raw leafy greens

Here are some examples of 1 cup and $1/2$ cup servings of vegetables from every subgroup.

VEGETABLE	AMOUNT THAT COUNTS AS 1 CUP	AMOUNT THAT COUNTS AS $1/2$ CUP
Dark Green		
Broccoli	1 cup chopped or florets	$1/2$ cup chopped or florets
Greens (collards, mustard greens, turnip greens, kale)	1 cup cooked	$1/2$ cup cooked
Raw Leafy Greens (spinach, romaine, watercress, endive, escarole)	1 cup cooked, 2 cups raw	$1/2$ cup cooked, 1 cup raw
Orange		
Carrots	2 medium, ~12 baby carrots	1 medium, ~6 baby carrots
Pumpkin	1 cup mashed, cooked	$1/2$ cup mashed, cooked
Sweet potato	1 large baked (~2" diameter)	$1/2$ large baked
Winter Squash (acorn, butternut, Hubbard)	1 cup cubed, cooked	$1/2$ acorn squash, baked = $3/4$ cup
Dry Beans and Peas		
Black Beans, Chickpeas, Kidney Beans, Pinto Beans, Soybeans, Black-Eyed Peas, etc.	1 cup whole or mashed, cooked	$1/2$ cup whole or mashed, cooked
Tofu	1 cup cubed, ~8 oz.	$1/2$ cup cubed, ~4 oz.
Starchy		
Corn, Yellow or White	1 large ear (8" to 9" long)	1 small ear (~ 6" long)
Green Peas	1 cup	$1/2$ cup
White Potatoes	1 medium, broiled or baked (2.5" to 3" diameter)	$1/2$ medium, broiled or baked
Other		
Bean Sprouts	1 cup cooked	$1/2$ cup cooked
Cauliflower	1 cup pieces or florets	$1/2$ cup pieces or florets
Celery	1 cup raw or cooked	$1/2$ cup raw or cooked
Cucumbers	1 cup raw	$1/2$ cup raw
Green or Wax Beans	1 cup cooked	$1/2$ cup cooked
Green or Red Peppers	1 large pepper (~3" diameter)	1 small pepper
Iceberg Lettuce	2 cups raw	1 cup raw
Mushrooms	1 cup raw or cooked	$1/2$ cup raw or cooked
Onions	1 cup raw or cooked	$1/2$ cup raw or cooked
Tomatoes	1 large (~3" diameter)	1 small (~2" diameter)
Summer Squash or Zucchini	1 cup cooked	$1/2$ cup cooked

Cups of vegetables I need a day: _____

STRATEGIES FOR EATING MORE VEGETABLES

- Readjust your environment and start keeping vegetables in your house. Utilize the crisper or vegetable drawer of your refrigerator, and stock it well.

- Buy fresh vegetables in season; they will be at their peak flavor, and they also may be less expensive.

- Keep frozen vegetables on hand for quick and easy cooking in the microwave.

- Consider convenience and try prewashed bags of salad, baby carrots and even butternut squash.

- When you buy your vegetables, wash them well, dry them off, wrap them in a paper towel and store them in a plastic bag in the refrigerator to maintain freshness.

- Plan some meals around a vegetarian dish, such as vegetable lasagna, homemade pizza or stir-fry.

- Spruce up your salads by adding other vegetables such as carrots, cucumber, corn or tomatoes; or add other tasty ingredients such as dried cranberries, nuts or seeds.

- Include cooked dry beans or peas in soups such as minestrone, chili or navy bean stew.

- Add some vegetable sweetness (such as shredded carrots or zucchini) to casseroles, quick breads and muffins.

- Grill bell peppers, squash, onions and tomatoes on kebobs.

- Bring a colorful relish tray to your next social event, and use low-fat dressing as a dip.

make at least half
your grains whole

Choose Often	Choose Occasionally	Choose Seldom
Whole-grain breads, bagels, tortillas, pitas, pasta and cereals; oats, brown rice, bulgur, low-fat whole-grain crackers, low-fat popcorn, pretzels	White bread and pasta that's not whole grain, baked corn tortillas, taco shells, baked chips, granola, regular crackers, fat-free cakes and cookies, biscuits, fig bars, angel food cake; French toast, waffles or pancakes made with whole grain	Fried chips, croissants, pastry, pies, doughnuts, sweet rolls, snack crackers with hydrogenated oils (trans fats), sweetened breakfast cereals, refined grain products prepared with cream, butter, sugar or cheese sauce

Bread and grain-based products have garnered a somewhat negative reputation over the years due to widespread misinformation through a mix of pop culture and bad science. This diverse group of nutritious and fiber-rich foods has been harpooned by numerous fad diets that accuse them of being the main culprit that leads to weight gain. However, foods made from grains and those products in their most wholesome forms not only protect from disease, but they also are a wise choice for anyone looking to manage their weight.

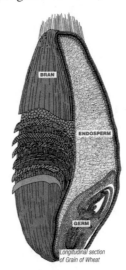

The key is to learn how to differentiate between refined grain products laden with sugar and fat and those that are made with whole grains. Whole grains maintain their nutritional value and integrity while leaving the extra calories and fat behind. In general, adults who exercise less than 30 minutes a day in addition to daily activities need 5 to 8 ounces of grains per day with 3 to 4 ounces of those being whole grains.

Grains are divided into two groups: *whole grains* and *refined grains*.

Longitudinal section of Grain of Wheat

(Image courtesy of the Wheat Foods Council)

Whole grains contain the entire grain kernel, which is made up of three parts: the bran, the germ and the endosperm. Your goal should be to make at least half your grain choices whole grains. Check the ingredients list for the words "whole grain" or "whole wheat" to decide if a product is truly whole grain. The word "whole" must be included, and it is best if you see "100% whole." One serving of whole grain is equal to 16 grams whole grain. Aim for at least 48 grams (or 3 servings) of whole grain each day.

Examples of whole grains include whole-wheat flour, graham flour, bulgur (cracked wheat), oatmeal/whole oats, whole cornmeal/whole-grain corn, whole rye, brown rice and wild rice.

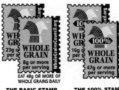

Images courtesy of the Whole Grains Council. Whole Grain Stamps are a trademark of Oldways Preservation Trust and the Whole Grains Council (www.wholegrainscouncil.org).

Refined grains have been milled—a process that removes the bran and the germ. Manufacturers do this to give grains a finer texture and improve their shelf life (the amount of time a product can be used before becoming rancid). Unfortunately, this process cheapens the product nutritionally because the dietary fiber, iron and many B vitamins (thiamin, riboflavin, niacin and folic acid) are stripped from the grain when the bran and germ are removed. One positive aspect of refined grains is that most are enriched, which means that certain B vitamins and iron are added back after processing. Unfortunately, fiber is not added back to enriched grains.

Examples of refined grains include white flour, de-germed cornmeal, white bread and white rice.

WHAT'S INCLUDED?

Any food made from wheat, rice, cornmeal, barley or another cereal grain is a grain product. Bread, pasta, oatmeal, breakfast cereals, crackers, tortillas and grits are examples of grain products.

WHAT COUNTS AS 1 OUNCE?

- 1 slice of bread
- 1 cup of ready-to-eat cereal (flakes or rounds)
- $1^1/_4$ cups of ready-to-eat cereal (puffs)
- $^1/_2$ cup of cooked rice, pasta or cereal

Unfortunately, the typical servings of most grain products have increased over the years. What used to be a typical bagel has more than tripled in size! Therefore, you must be conscious of your portions by reading labels (look for ounces per serving) and estimating portion size using visual cues. Here are a few examples:

- A small bagel or roll should be around the size of a hockey puck.
- A medium-sized potato should resemble the size of a computer mouse or a woman's fist.
- A half cup of pasta or rice would fill the size of a rounded handful.

Most of the grain products you eat will not come in 1-ounce servings. That is perfectly fine. However, you need to begin learning how much you're actually eating when you pick up that bagel on the way to work, for example. The following chart lists specific amounts of common foods that count as 1 ounce toward your daily recommended intake as well as typical portions that you find today. Each item is also denoted as "whole" or "refined" with examples of whole-grain and refined-grain choices for appropriate items.

ITEM	EXAMPLES OF WHOLE VERSUS REFINED GRAINS	AMOUNT THAT COUNTS AS 1 OUNCE	TYPICAL PORTIONS AND OUNCE EQUIVALENTS
Bagel	Whole: 100% whole-grain Refined: plain or egg	$1/2$ minibagel	1 large bagel = 4 oz. equivalents
Biscuit	Whole: whole-wheat flour Refined: white flour	1 small (2" diameter)	1 large (3" diameter) = 2 oz. equivalents
Bread	Whole: 100% whole-rye Refined: white, wheat, French, sourdough	1 regular slice 1 small slice French 4 snack-sized slices rye bread	2 regular slices = 2 oz. equivalents
Bulgur/Cracked Wheat	Whole	$1/2$ cup cooked	
Cornbread	Whole: whole-grain cornmeal Refined: de-germed cornmeal	1 small piece ($2^1/_2$" x $1^1/_4$" x $1^1/_4$")	1 medium piece ($2^1/_2$" x $2^1/_2$" x $1^1/_4$") = 2 oz. equivalents
Crackers	Whole: 100% whole-wheat, rye Refined: saltines, snack crackers unless denoted as whole-grain	5 whole-wheat crackers, 2 rye crispbreads, 7 square or round crackers	
English Muffins	Whole: whole-wheat Refined: plain, raisin	$1/2$ muffin	1 muffin = 2 oz. equivalents
Muffins	Whole: whole-wheat Refined: bran, corn	1 small ($2^1/_2$" diameter)	1 large ($3^1/_2$" diameter) = 3 oz. equivalents
Oatmeal	Whole	$1/2$ cup cooked, 1 packet instant, 1 oz. dry (regular or quick)	
Pancakes	Whole: whole-wheat, buckwheat Refined: plain, buttermilk	1 pancake ($4^1/_2$" diameter)	3 pancakes ($4^1/_2$" diameter) = 3 oz. equivalents
Pasta	Whole: whole-wheat Refined: enriched, durum	$1/2$ cup cooked, 1 oz. dry	1 cup cooked = 2 oz. equivalents
Popcorn	Whole	3 cups, popped	1 regular microwave bag, popped = 4 oz. equivalents
Ready-to-Eat Cereal	Whole: toasted oat, whole-wheat flakes Refined: corn flakes, puffed rice	1 cup flakes or rounds, $1^1/_4$ cup puffed	
Rice	Whole: brown, wild Refined: white, enriched, polished	$1/2$ cup cooked, 1 oz. dry	1 cup cooked = 2 oz. equivalents
Tortillas	Whole: whole-wheat, whole-grain corn Refined: flour, de-germed corn	1 small flour tortilla (6" diameter), 1 corn tortilla (6" diameter)	1 large tortilla (12" diameter) = 4 oz. equivalents

Ounces of grain products I need a day: _____

HEALTH BENEFITS FROM EATING WHOLE GRAINS

Grains provide many nutrients that are essential for the health and maintenance of our bodies. Whole grains are important sources of fiber, several B vitamins (thiamin, riboflavin, niacin and folic acid) and minerals (iron, magnesium and selenium). Eating a diet rich in whole grains protects against some chronic diseases such as coronary heart disease as well as gastrointestinal conditions such as constipation and diverticulosis.

Again we learn how foods are greater than the sum of their parts. The inherent balance of nutrients in each food group supplies certain benefits that cannot be met by other groups or by supplements alone. Variety in your diet is essential for proper nutrition and protection from boredom!

STRATEGIES FOR EATING MORE WHOLE GRAINS

Read the Label

- More often choose foods that name at least one whole-grain ingredient first on the label's ingredient list. Examples include but are not limited to brown rice, bulgur, graham flour, oatmeal, whole-grain corn, whole oats, whole rye, whole wheat and wild rice.

- Be careful! Foods labeled with the words "multigrain," "stone-ground," "100% wheat," "cracked wheat," "seven-grain" or "bran" are usually not whole-grain products. Always look for the word "whole."

- Color is not a reliable indication of whether a product is whole grain. Molasses and other added ingredients can alter the color.

- Read the Nutrition Facts Panel (see "Understanding the Nutrition Facts Panel" in this guide), and choose products with a higher percentage Daily Value (%DV) for fiber, as it is a good clue to the amount of whole grain in a product.

- Look for terms that indicate added sugars ("sucrose," "high-fructose corn syrup," "honey" and "molasses") and oils ("partially hydrogenated vegetable oils") that add extra calories. Most often choose foods with fewer added sugars, fats or oils.

- Most sodium in our food supply comes from packaged foods. Even breads vary in sodium content, so use the NFP and choose foods with a lower %DV for sodium. Foods with less than 140 milligrams of sodium per serving can be labeled "low sodium" foods.

Meals and Snacks

- Substitute whole-grain products for refined products when preparing meals (whole-wheat pasta, whole-wheat pizza crust or brown rice).

- Try using rolled oats or crushed whole-grain cereal as breading for baked chicken, fish or eggplant Parmesan.

- Add some barley to your vegetable soup or stews.

- Use whole-grain flour or oat flour for up to half of the flour in pancake, waffle, muffin or other flour-based recipes.

- Whole-grain cereals and popcorn with little or no added salt make tasty and wholesome snacks!

get your
calcium-rich foods!

Choose Often	Choose Occasionally	Choose Seldom
Skim milk, 1% milk and buttermilk, nonfat and low-fat yogurt, nonfat frozen yogurt; part-skim, low-fat and fat-free cheese; low-fat and fat-free cottage cheese, soy milk, soy cheese	2% milk, 2% cheese, 4% cottage cheese, light cream cheese, light sour cream, low-fat sherbet, processed cheese spreads, light nondairy whipped cream	whole milk, regular cheese, cream, half-and-half, most nondairy creamers, whipped cream, full-fat nondairy whipped cream, full-fat cream cheese, full-fat sour cream, full-fat ice cream, full-fat yogurt

Studies have shown that "milking your diet" daily with 3 cups of low-fat milk or other low-fat dairy products in addition to eating a reduced-calorie diet supports healthy weight loss. Simply stated, diets that include milk products tend to have a higher overall nutritional quality. Compared to the sugar-sweetened beverages that many Americans choose, milk is a healthier option full of protein, vitamins and minerals. You don't lose nutrients when you choose fat-free (skim) or low fat (1%) milk; you only lose the fat!

WHAT'S INCLUDED?

All fluid milk products and many foods made from milk are considered part of this food group. Foods made from milk that retain their calcium content are included, but foods made from milk that have little to no calcium, such as cream cheese and butter, are not. Some commonly eaten choices in the milk group are plain milk, flavored milk (chocolate or strawberry), lactose-reduced and lactose-free milks, puddings made with milk, frozen yogurt, hard cheeses (cheddar, mozzarella, Swiss and Parmesan), soft cheeses (ricotta and cottage), processed cheeses (American), and yogurt.

Whole milk and many cheeses—and products made from them (full-fat ice cream, for example)—are high in saturated fat. To help keep blood cholesterol levels healthy and to promote weight loss, limit the amount of these foods you eat to very little.

WHAT COUNTS AS 1 CUP?

- 1 cup milk
- 1 cup yogurt
- $1^1/_2$ ounces natural cheese
- 2 ounces processed cheese

ITEM (most often choose fat-free or low-fat)	AMOUNT THAT COUNTS AS 1 CUP	TYPICAL PORTIONS AND CUP EQUIVALENTS
Milk	1 cup, 1 half-pint container, $^1/_2$ cup evaporated milk	
Yogurt	1 regular container (1 cup or 8 oz.)	1 small container (6 oz.) = $^3/_4$ cup; snack-sized container (4 oz.) = $^1/_2$ cup
Cheese	$1^1/_2$ oz. hard cheese (cheddar, mozzarella, Swiss, Parmesan), $^1/_3$ cup shredded cheese, 2 oz. processed cheese (American), $^1/_2$ cup ricotta cheese, 2 cups cottage cheese	1 slice of processed cheese is equivalent to $^1/_3$ cup milk
Milk-Based Desserts	1 cup pudding made with milk, 1 cup frozen yogurt	

Cups of milk and/or milk products I need a day: _____

HEALTH BENEFITS FROM EATING MILK AND MILK PRODUCTS

Foods in the milk group provide nutrients that are vital for our body's health and maintenance, such as calcium, potassium, vitamin D and protein.

- Milk products are the primary source for calcium in American diets. Calcium is used for building strong bones and teeth as well as for protecting against lost bone mass (osteoporosis).

- The potassium in milk may help to maintain healthy blood pressure.

- Vitamin D functions in the body to maintain proper levels of calcium and phosphorus, which help to build and maintain bones.

- Fat-free and low-fat milk and milk products provide a lot of nutrition with little or no solid fat, which helps to maintain caloric balance and promote weight loss.

NONDAIRY ITEM	CALCIUM CONTENT (mg)
Orange juice, calcium fortified, 1 cup	351
Sardines, Atlantic, in oil, drained, 3 oz.	325
Soymilk, calcium fortified, 1 cup	299
Tofu, firm, prepared with nigari, $1/_2$ cup	253
Blackstrap molasses, 1 tablespoon	200
Pink salmon, canned with bone, 3 oz.	181
Collards, cooked from frozen, $1/_2$ cup	178
Spinach, cooked from frozen, $1/_2$ cup	145
Soybeans, green, cooked, $1/_2$ cup	130
Turnip greens, cooked from frozen, $1/_2$ cup	125
Ocean perch, Atlantic, cooked, 3 oz.	116
Oatmeal, plain and flavored, instant, fortified, 1 packet prepared with water	109-187
Cowpeas or blackeyes, cooked, $1/_2$ cup	106
White beans, canned, $1/_2$ cup	96
Kale, cooked from frozen, $1/_2$ cup	90
Okra, cooked from frozen, $1/_2$ cup	88
Soybeans, mature, cooked, $1/_2$ cup	88
Blue crab, canned, 3 oz.	86
Beet greens, cooked from fresh, $1/_2$ cup	82
Bok choy, Chinese cabbage, cooked from fresh, $1/_2$ cup	79
Clams, canned, 3 oz.	78
Dandelion greens, cooked from fresh, $1/_2$ cup	74
Rainbow trout, farmed, cooked, 3 oz.	73

(Nutrient values from *Agricultural Research Service (ARS) Nutrient Database for Standard Release, Release 20*)

STRATEGIES FOR EATING MORE MILK PRODUCTS

- Include fat-free or low-fat milk as a beverage at meals.

- If you usually drink whole milk or 2% milk, switch gradually to the low-fat (1%) or no-fat (skim) option.

- If you drink lattes or cappuccinos, ask for fat-free milk to be used.

- Add fat-free milk or low-fat milk instead of water when cooking oatmeal and hot cereals.

- Use fat-free or low-fat milk when making condensed cream soups.

- Have a low-fat or fat-free yogurt as a snack.

- Make a yogurt-based dip for fruit as a snack.

- Make fruit-yogurt smoothies in the blender.

- For dessert, try chocolate or French-vanilla pudding made with fat-free or low-fat milk.

- Try topping casseroles, soups, stews or vegetables with shredded low-fat (part-skim) cheese.

DEALING WITH LACTOSE INTOLERANCE

If you are lactose intolerant, lactose-free and lower-lactose products are available in most grocery stores. These include hard cheeses and yogurt as well as liquid milk. Also, enzyme preparations can be added to milk to lower the lactose content.

Calcium-fortified foods and beverages such as soy beverages and orange juice may provide calcium but may not provide the other nutrients found in milk and milk products. Check with your doctor about possibly taking a calcium supplement if you are lactose intolerant and do not think you are obtaining at least 1,000 milligrams of calcium from the nondairy food sources of calcium shown on the previous page. Both calcium content and bioavailability should be considered when selecting dietary sources of calcium. Some plant foods have calcium that is well absorbed, but the large quantity of plant foods that would be needed to provide as much calcium as in a glass of milk may be unachievable for many. For comparison's sake, 1 cup of skim or low-fat fluid milk with added vitamin A provides approximately 300 milligrams of calcium.

go lean with protein!

Choose Often	Choose Occasionally	Choose Seldom
Lean cuts of beef and pork, extra-lean ground beef (90% to 95% lean), poultry without skin, dried beans and peas, lentils, tofu, egg whites, egg substitutes; baked, broiled, grilled or steamed fish; tuna canned with water	Lean ground beef (85% to 90% lean), whole eggs cooked without fat, fish sticks (baked), tuna canned in oil, poultry with skin, ham, Canadian bacon, chicken nuggets (baked), turkey hot dogs, nuts, nut butters	Prime-grade meats, ribs, duck, goose, dark poultry meat, regular ground beef (75% to 85% lean), bacon, sausage, pepperoni, whole eggs cooked with fat, bologna, salami, hot dogs, ribs, organ meats; fried fish, chicken or beef

While most Americans have no problem eating enough protein every day (some of us get way too much, actually), we do seem to have a hard time choosing *quality* protein-rich foods. By choosing meat that is low in saturated fat and cholesterol, as well as incorporating vegetarian sources of protein into your diet, you can provide your body with the nutrients it needs for maintenance and repair but save yourself the added fat, cholesterol and calories.

WHAT'S INCLUDED?

Lean meats, poultry, fish, eggs, dry beans and peas, nuts and seeds all count toward meeting the meat and beans group goals. Dry beans and peas are vegetarian alternatives to meat and are included in both this and the vegetable group. Most meat and poultry choices should be lean or low-fat and cooked using healthy methods such as baking, broiling or grilling with little added fat or salt. Fish, nuts and seeds contain healthy unsaturated oils (as opposed to saturated fat), so frequently choose these foods. Most adults who exercise less than 30 minutes a day in addition to daily activities need 5 to 6-1/2 ounces of meat and beans per day.

WHAT COUNTS AS 1 OUNCE?

- 1 ounce of meat, poultry or fish
- $1/4$ cup cooked dry beans
- 1 egg
- 1 tablespoon peanut butter
- $1/2$ ounce nuts or seeds

ITEM	AMOUNT THAT COUNTS AS 1 OUNCE	TYPICAL PORTIONS AND OUNCE EQUIVALENTS
Meats	1 oz. cooked lean beef, lean pork or ham	1 small steak (eye of round or filet) = $3^1/2$–4 oz. equivalents 1 small lean hamburger = 2-3 oz. equivalents
Poultry	1 oz. cooked chicken or turkey without skin, 1 sandwich slice of turkey ($4^1/2$" x $2^1/2$" x $1/8$")	1 small chicken breast half = 3 oz. equivalents $1/2$ Cornish game hen = 4 oz. equivalents
Fish	1 oz. cooked fish or shellfish	1 can tuna = 3-4 oz. equivalents 1 salmon steak = 4-6 oz. equivalents 1 small trout = 3 oz. equivalents
Eggs	1 egg	3-egg omelet = 3 oz. equivalents
Nuts and Seeds	$1/2$ oz. nuts (12 almonds, 24 pistachios or 7 walnut halves), $1/2$ oz. seeds (pumpkin, sunflower or squash seeds, hulled and roasted), 1 tablespoon of peanut or almond butter	1 oz. nuts or seeds = 2 oz. equivalents
Dry Beans and Peas	$1/4$ cup cooked dry beans (such as black, kidney, pinto or white beans), $1/4$ cup cooked dry peas (chickpeas, cowpeas, lentils or split peas), $1/4$ cup baked beans, $1/4$ cup refried beans, $1/4$ cup tofu (about 2 oz.), 1 oz. cooked tempeh, $1/4$ cup roasted soybeans, 2 tablespoons hummus, 1 falafel patty (4 oz.)	1 cup split pea, lentil or bean soup = 2 oz. equivalents 1 soy or bean burger patty = 2 oz. equivalents

Ounce-equivalents of meat and bean products I need a day: _____

WHY GO LEAN?

Diets high in saturated fats raise "bad" cholesterol levels in the blood. The "bad" cholesterol is LDL (low-density lipoprotein) cholesterol. High LDL cholesterol, in turn, increases the risk for coronary heart disease. Some food choices in this group are high in saturated fat. These include fatty cuts of beef, pork and lamb; regular (75% to 85% lean) ground beef; regular sausages, hot dogs and bacon; some luncheon meats such as regular bologna and salami; and some poultry such as duck. To help keep blood cholesterol levels healthy, limit the amount of these foods you eat.

Diets high in cholesterol can also raise LDL cholesterol levels in the blood. Cholesterol is only found in foods from animal sources, and some foods in this meat and beans group are high in cholesterol. These high-cholesterol foods include egg yolks (egg whites are cholesterol-free) and organ meats such as liver and giblets. Again, eat these foods in moderation to help keep blood cholesterol levels healthy.

Fatty cuts of meat not only raise cholesterol, but they also can raise your calorie intake for the day. A high intake of fats makes it difficult to avoid consuming more calories than are required to maintain or lose weight, so be sure to choose lean meats most often.

FOCUS ON FATTY ACIDS

Varying choices and including fish, nuts and seeds in meals can boost your intake of monounsaturated fatty acids (MUFAs) and polyunsaturated fatty acids (PUFAs). Most fat in the diet should come from MUFAs and PUFAs. Some of the PUFAs are essential for health—the body cannot create them from other fats. Some fish (such as salmon, trout and herring) are high in omega-3 fatty acids, a type of PUFA. The omega-3 fatty acids in fish are commonly known as EPA and DHA. There is some limited evidence that suggests eating fish rich in EPA and DHA may reduce the risk for cardiovascular disease. Some nuts and seeds (like flax and walnuts) are excellent sources of essential fatty acids, and some (such as sunflower seeds, almonds and hazelnuts) are good sources of vitamin E.

HEALTH BENEFITS FROM EATING LEAN PROTEIN

Nutrients supplied by foods in this group include protein, B vitamins (niacin, thiamin, riboflavin and B_6), vitamin E, iron, magnesium and zinc.

- Proteins function as building blocks for bones, muscles, cartilage, skin and blood. They are also building blocks for enzymes, hormones and vitamins. Proteins are one of three nutrients that provide calories (the others are fat and carbohydrates).

- B vitamins found in this food group serve a variety of functions in the body. They help the body release energy, play a vital role in the function of the nervous system, aid in the formation of red blood cells, and help build tissues.

- Vitamin E is an antioxidant that helps protect vitamin A and essential fatty acids from cell oxidation.

- Iron is used to carry oxygen in the blood. Many teenage girls and women in their childbearing years have iron-deficiency anemia. They should eat foods high in heme iron (meats) or eat other non-heme iron-containing foods along with foods rich in vitamin C, which can improve absorption of non-heme iron.

- Magnesium is used in building bones and in releasing energy from muscles.

- Zinc is necessary for biochemical reactions and helps the immune system function properly.

STRATEGIES FOR EATING MORE LEAN PROTEIN

Start with a Lean Choice

- The leanest cuts of beef include round steaks and roasts (round eye, top round, bottom round and round tip), top loin, top sirloin, chuck shoulder and arm roasts.

- The leanest cuts of pork include pork loin, tenderloin, center loin and ham.

- Choose extra-lean ground beef. Look for labels that say 90% lean or even 93% or 95% lean.

- Buy skinless chicken or remove the skin before eating.

- Choose lean turkey, roast beef, ham or low-fat luncheon meats for sandwiches instead of luncheon meats with more fat (like regular bologna or salami).

Keep It Lean

- Trim away all visible fat from meat before cooking and poultry before eating.

- Broil, grill, roast, poach or boil meat, poultry or fish instead of frying.

- Drain off any fat that appears during cooking.

- Rinse ground beef after cooking it.

- Prepare beans and peas without adding any fat.

- If you prepare a sauce to complement your meat, make a low-fat sauce.

Vary Your Protein Choices

- Try to eat fish three times a week. Look for fish rich in omega-3 fatty acids such as wild salmon, trout and herring.

- Make some meals vegetarian but still rich in protein by using dry beans, peas or nuts. Some examples include chili with kidney beans or pinto beans; stir-fried tofu; split pea, lentil, minestrone or white bean soup; baked beans; and black bean quesadillas or enchiladas. You can also add garbanzo or kidney beans to your salad; grill up a veggie or garden burger; go Greek with hummus on pita bread; use pine nuts in pesto sauce for your favorite pasta; add slivered almonds to steamed veggies; and choose nuts as a snack or include them in salads or main dishes. (When you use nuts, replace meat or poultry with them to stay within your calorie range.)

choose
healthy oils!

Choose Often	Choose Occasionally	Choose Seldom
Olive oil, canola oil, peanut oil, fat-free mayonnaise	Safflower, corn, soybean, sesame and sunflower oils; mayonnaise made with canola oil; light or reduced-fat mayonnaise, lower-fat salad dressings, trans fat-free margarine	Butter, lard, beef tallow, bacon fat, regular mayonnaise, full-fat salad dressings, shortening, palm kernel and coconut oils, stick margarine or shortening made with hydrogenated oil and containing trans fats

Healthy oils? Yes, that's right! Some types of oil, a liquid fat, can actually be good for you when used appropriately! First, you have to consider the *quality* of the fat you eat. The level of quality for a fat is determined by whether or not it's saturated (solid) or unsaturated (liquid). Your goal is to choose foods with unsaturated fats most, if not all, of the time. Unsaturated fats include both monounsaturated fatty acids (MUFAs) and polyunsaturated fats (PUFAs). By choosing unsaturated fats, you lower your intake of saturated and trans fat but still provide your body with the essential fatty acids and the vitamin E it needs.

Second, you have to remember that *quantity counts*! With fats providing 9 calories per gram (think 120 calories per tablespoon of vegetable oil), you have to use them sparingly and most often choose low-fat foods from every group in the pyramid. For someone who exercises less than 30 minutes a day in addition to daily activities, 5 to 7 teaspoons of oil are sufficient. *This amount includes the oils contained in foods, not in addition to them!* (For an in-depth look at fats, refer to "The Facts on Fats" in *Simple Ideas for Healthy Living* in your Member's Kit.)

WHAT'S INCLUDED?

As far as their content, all solid fats and liquid oils are a mixture of MUFAs and PUFAs. However, solid fats contain a higher distribution of saturated fatty acids than oils, and oils contain a higher distribution of unsaturated fatty acids than solid fats. Solid fats also include trans fatty acids.

Saturated fats, trans fats and dietary cholesterol tend to raise the "bad" (LDL) choles-terol levels in the blood, which in turn increases the risk for heart disease. To lower this risk and even work to prevent it, replace foods containing saturated fats, trans fats and choles-terol with foods higher in unsaturated fats.

WHAT ARE OILS?

Oils are fats that are liquid at room temperature. Most oils are high in monounsaturated or polyunsaturated fats, and low in saturated fats. Oils come from many different plants and from some fish, and some oils are used mainly for flavor, such as walnut oil and sesame oil. Oils from plant sources (vegetable and nut oils) do not contain any cholesterol. A few plant oils (including coconut oils and palm kernel oil), however, are high in saturated fat and for nutritional purposes should be considered to be solid fats. Some common plant oils are canola, corn, cottonseed, olive, safflower, soybean, sunflower and flaxseed oils.

A number of foods are naturally high in oils; these include nuts, olives, some fish (like salmon, mackerel and herring) and avocados.

Foods that are mainly oil include mayonnaise, certain salad dressings and soft (tub or squeeze) margarine with no trans fats. Be sure to read the Nutrition Facts Panel (NFP) on margarines, and choose ones with no trans fat.

WHAT ARE SOLID FATS?

Solid fats are fats that are solid at room temperature, like butter or shortening. Solid fats come from many animal foods and can be made from vegetable oils through a process called hydrogenation. Some common solid fats are butter, beef fat (tallow and suet), chicken fat, pork fat (lard), stick margarine and most shortenings.

A number of foods are high in solid fats, such as many cheeses, creams, ice creams, well-marbled cuts of meats, regular ground beef, bacon, sausages, poultry skin and many baked goods (such as cookies, crackers, donuts and croissants).

WHAT COUNTS AS 1 TEASPOON?

Because most Americans consume more than enough oil in the foods they eat, additional servings of oil are not required. In fact, most of us are consuming way too much fat (and the calories that come with it). Even if you are consuming a relatively low-fat diet, if it is rich in variety, *you are getting enough fat.* Foods that often take care of our oil quota for the day include nuts, some fish, foods cooked with oil, and salad dressings. Note that these foods contain mostly unsaturated, or healthy, oils, which contribute quality fat to our diet. However, this means that your daily allotment of oil, or the quantity you need to stay within your calorie range, is accomplished by eating a varied diet. In other words, you don't need 6 extra teaspoons of oil a day. Those 6 teaspoons are already contained in many of the foods you should be eating. To help you understand how much oil exists in some common foods, review the table below.

FOODS RICH IN OILS	SERVING SIZE	AMOUNT OF OIL
Margarine, soft, trans-fat-free	1 tablespoon	$2^1/_2$ teaspoons
Mayonnaise	1 tablespoon	$2^1/_2$ teaspoons
Mayonnaise-type salad dressing	1 tablespoon	1 teaspoon
Italian dressing	2 tablespoons	2 teaspoons
Thousand Island dressing	2 tablespoons	$2^1/_2$ teaspoons
Olives, ripe, canned	4 large	$^1/_2$ teaspoon
Avocado*	$^1/_2$ medium	3 teaspoons
Peanut butter**	2 tablespoons	4 teaspoons
Peanuts, dry roasted**	1 oz.	3 teaspoons
Mixed nuts, dry roasted**	1 oz.	3 teaspoons
Cashews, dry roasted**	1 oz.	3 teaspoons
Almonds, dry roasted**	1 oz.	3 teaspoons
Hazelnuts**	1 oz.	4 teaspoons
Sunflower seeds**	1 oz.	3 teaspoons

* Avocados are part of the fruit group
** Nuts, nut butters, and seeds are part of the meat and beans group

understanding the nutrition facts panel

T here is more information to help you choose the best foods for health available to you on food and beverage packaging than you probably realize. The Nutrition Facts Panel (NFP) provides all the information you need to know, and it's easy to learn how to read this label so that you can become a better educated and more health-conscious consumer. The NFP provides information on an array of factors that qualify a serving of a beverage or food as something to choose or stay away from.[1]

INGREDIENTS

Ingredients are listed on the NFP in order from the greatest amount included in the food or drink to the least amount. For example, if you see sugar or one of its other names listed at the beginning or close to the beginning of the ingredients list, then you know that the food or drink you're looking at is predominantly high in sugar.

Based upon what you see on this list, you can make an educated guess about which food groups the product includes. Keep alert to heart-healthy ingredients such as whole-wheat flour, soy and oats; and monounsaturated fats such as olive, canola or peanut oils, which promote heart health. Likewise, use food labels to detect unhealthy ingredients such as hydrogenated or partially hydrogenated oil.

The bottom line? Look for products with the fewest ingredients—and the ones with ingredients that you can actually pronounce!

Nutrition Facts

Serving Size 3 oz (85g)
Serving Per Container 1

Amount Per Serving

Calories 180	Calories from Fat 90

	% Daily Value*
Total Fat 10g	**15%**
Saturated Fat 40g	**20%**
Trans Fat 0.5g	
Cholesterol 70mg	**23%**
Sodium 60mg	**3%**
Total Carbohydrate 0g	**0%**
Dietary Fiber 0g	**0%**
Sugars 0g	
Protein 22g	

Vitamin A 0%	•	Vitamin C 0%	
Calcium 2%	•	Iron 15%	

*Percent Daily Values are based on a 2,000 calorie diet. Your daily values may be higher or lower depending on your caloric needs:

		Calories:	2,000	2,500
Total Fat	Less than		65g	80g
Saturated Fat	Less than		20g	25g
Cholesterol	Less than		300mg	300mg
Sodiuum	Less than		2,400mg	2,400mg
Total Carbohydrate			300g	375g
Dietary Fiber			25g	30g

Calories per gram:
Fat 9 • Carbohydrate 4 • Protein 4

(Image courtesy of the FDA)

SERVING SIZE

Don't fall into the sly trap of portion distortion! Educate yourself and learn what a serving is for the product you're considering. The Food and Drug Administration (FDA) determines the serving size described on the food labels of many foods. The FDA uses a "usual serving" or "reference amount."[2] This makes it easier to compare different brands of a food, because the serving sizes will be the same. This also assures that a food cannot be called low-fat when a very small serving size is used. All the information on a food label is based on the serving size given, which may be smaller than you think! And don't expect manufacturers to make it easy for you. Some convenience items, for instance, come two to a package, but the label says that one serving is *one* of the two items, not both! (More about portion distortion in the next article in this guide.)

CALORIES

Make calories count! Look at the calories *per serving* on the label and compare them with the nutrients they offer. Go for the biggest nutritional bang for your calories as well as for your buck. Choosing *nutrient*-dense foods as opposed to *calorie*-dense foods will not only help you monitor your weight but will also ensure that you get what your body really needs—the proper nutrition. Calories derived from fat are indicated by the *number* of calories from fat, *not* by the percentage. If you want to determine the percentage, divide the calories from fat by the total calories and multiply by 100. On average, choose more foods with 35 percent or less of the calories derived from fat. Not every food you eat has to be less than 35 percent fat—just the overall balance of foods you eat.

PERCENTAGE DAILY VALUE (%DV)

Percentage Daily Values are based on a 2,000-calorie diet and are to be used as a frame of reference. Your daily values may be higher or lower, depending on your individual needs. However, this section does give you some valuable information regarding the *proportion* of nutrients in a food and whether a food is high or low in nutrients. Foods that have 20% DV or more of a nutrient are high. Foods that have 5% DV or less are low. Use this information, not only to help you limit those nutrients you want to cut back on (fat, saturated fat, cholesterol and sodium), but also to increase those nutrients you need to consume in greater amounts (fiber, vitamins A and C, calcium and iron).

DAILY VALUES

A footnote at the bottom of most food labels provides the suggested daily values of certain nutrients usually based on two calorie levels: 2,000 calories and 2,500 calories. Again, these numbers are a frame of reference for the average individual eating either 2,000 or 2,500 calories. Notice which nutrients stay the same regardless of calorie level.

Nutrient	Recommendation	2,000 kcal	2,500 kcal
Total Fat	Less than	65 g	80 g
Saturated Fat	Less than	20 g	25 g
Cholesterol	Less than	300 mg	300 mg
Sodium	Less than	2,400 mg	2,400 mg
Total Carbohydrate	At least	300 g	375 g
Dietary Fiber	At least	25 g	30 g

TOTAL FAT

Total fat is provided in grams and %DV. Look at your calorie goals, and then choose to monitor your fat intake by either total fat grams or by %DV; 20 to 35 percent of your diet should come from healthy fats like mono- and polyunsaturated fats and oils (such as fish, vegetable oils, nuts and seeds). Remember, just because a food is "low-fat," "reduced-fat" or "light" does not always mean the food is low in calories—or sugar for that matter. Look at the big picture and consider all the major factors of whether a food is truly a healthy choice or not.

SATURATED FAT

Knowing the breakdown of fat in a particular food is as important as knowing the total amount of fat. Saturated fat is one of the worst things for your health. Compare the labels on similar foods and try to choose foods that have 5% DV or less or have 2 grams or less of saturated fat. The American Heart Association (AHA) recommends that saturated fat make up 7 percent or less of your total calories.[3] For a person on a diet of 1,600 calories, that equals 112 calories (1,600 calories × 0.07), or 12.4 grams, of saturated fat per day (112 calories ÷ 9). Those grams of saturated fat can add up really fast if you're not careful!

TRANS FAT

Thankfully, the harm of consuming trans fat is public knowledge. All the publicity it has received will hopefully lead to reduced intake of this LDL-raising, HDL-lowering, atherosclerosis-promoting fat! As of January 1, 2006, food manufacturers were required to list trans fat on their labels. The threshold for a "0g trans fat" product is 0.49 grams trans fat.[4] What that means is that some trans fat (albeit only 0.0 to 0.49 grams) may actually be in a product advertised as containing "0g trans fat." What is a health-conscious consumer to do? Scroll down the ingredients list again, and avoid products containing "hydrogenated" or "partially hydrogenated" anything!

CHOLESTEROL

You will want to keep your consumption of cholesterol as low as possible. Your liver makes enough cholesterol on its own; you really don't need much from your diet at all. The current adult recommendation for dietary cholesterol is no more than 300 milligrams per day. Cholesterol is found in organs and other meats, poultry, dairy products, shellfish and egg yolks. Foods of plant origin (vegetables, fruits, grains, nuts and seeds) contain no cholesterol. Fat content is not necessarily a good measurement of cholesterol content. For example, liver and other organ meats are low in fat but very high in cholesterol.

SODIUM

Salt (sodium chloride, or NaCl) contains sodium (Na); 2,400 milligrams of sodium is equal to about only 1 teaspoon of salt! Does that shock you? High sodium intake is linked to high blood pressure and hypertension. Look for labels that read "sodium-free" or "low-sodium." Foods that are "low" in sodium contain no more than 5% DV, or around 140 milligrams or less per serving. In 2004, the National Academy of Sciences Institute of Medicine came out with a new dietary reference intake (DRI) for sodium that differs from some food labels. ("Dietary Reference Intake" or DRI is a new term that replaces "U.S. Recommended Daily Allowance" [RDA]. The percentages that a food contributes to the RDI for certain nutrients, or the %DV, are listed on the food label.) The recommendation for adults is a daily sodium consumption of between 1,200 and 1,500 milligrams per day, with a tolerable upper limit of 2,300 milligrams (as opposed to the previous upper limit of 2,400 milligrams).[5] Intakes over the upper limit are considered to be harmful to your health. (One teaspoon of table salt is approximately 6,000 milligrams; however, table salt is made up of 40 percent sodium and 60 percent chloride, so it yields approximately 2,400 milligrams of sodium (40 percent of 6,000 milligrams).

FIBER

The daily adult goal for fiber intake is 21 grams to 38 grams depending on your age. With so many yummy foods to choose from (foods rich in whole grains, fruits and vegetables), you can achieve that goal painlessly, but you had better get started! Fiber lowers cholesterol, keeps your gut happy and fills you up!

SUGAR

Foods with added sugars provide calories but few essential nutrients. One important thing to keep in mind when reading a food label is that the naturally occurring sugars in some foods (dairy and fruits) are included in the total grams of sugar listed for a product. Therefore, a food seemingly high in sugar may contain *few* added sugars (added during processing and preparation). Again, this is where reading the ingredients list comes in handy. The added sugars (or caloric sweeteners) you want to steer clear of usually come in one (or more) of these forms: brown sugar, corn sweetener, corn syrup, dextrose, fructose, fruit juice concentrates, glucose, high-fructose corn syrup, honey, invert sugar, lactose, maltose, malt syrup, molasses, raw sugar, sucrose, sugar or syrup.

Plain Yogurt

INGREDIENTS: CULTURED PASTEURIZED GRADE A NONFAT MILK, WHEY PROTEIN CONCENTRATE, PECTIN, CARRAGEENAN.

Fruit Yogurt

INGREDIENTS: CULTURED GRADE A REDUCED FAT MILK, APPLES, HIGH FRUCTOSE CORN SYRUP, CINNAMON, NUTMEG, NATURAL FLAVORS, AND PECTIN.

VITAMINS AND MINERALS

Your goal is to consume 100 percent of each of the vitamin and mineral nutrients daily. The specific vitamins and minerals listed on the food label are those that are most vulnerable to deficiency in the United States. Many other vitamins and minerals not listed are just as important but are usually consumed in adequate amounts. By selecting a variety of nutrient-dense foods, you can achieve 100-percent intake of most vitamins and minerals and don't need to use supplements.

UNDERSTANDING NUTRITION AND HEALTH CLAIMS

When it comes to health and nutrition claims, you *can* believe what you read. Food makers must meet strict government guidelines to use terms such as "low fat" or "reduced sodium" or to make health claims about heart disease, cancer or other diseases. Only health claims that are supported by scientific evidence and approved by the FDA are allowed. Refer to the chart of terms and definitions below.

TERM	DEFINITION
Calorie free	5 or fewer calories per serving
Low calorie	40 or fewer calories per serving
Fat free	Less than $1/2$ (0.5) gram of total fat per serving
Low fat	3 or fewer grams of total fat per serving
Saturated fat free	Less than $1/2$ (0.5) gram of saturated fat per serving
Low saturated fat	Less than 1 gram of saturated fat per serving
Zero trans fat	Contains 0 to 0.49 grams of trans fat per serving
Cholesterol free	2 or fewer milligrams of cholesterol and 2 or fewer grams of saturated fat per serving
Low cholesterol	20 or fewer milligrams of cholesterol and 2 or fewer grams of saturated fat per serving
Sodium free	5 or fewer milligrams of sodium per serving
Low sodium	140 or fewer milligrams of sodium per serving
Very low sodium	35 or fewer milligrams of sodium per serving
Sugar free	Less than $1/2$ (0.5) gram of sugar per serving
No sugar added	No sugars added during processing or packaging
Light, or Lite	$1/3$ less calories or 50 percent less of a nutrient such as fat, sodium or sugar than the regular or reference food
Reduced	25 percent less calories, fat, saturated fat, cholesterol, sodium or sugar than the regular or reference food; words such as "lower" and "fewer" may also be used
Lean	10 or fewer grams of fat, 4.5 or fewer grams of saturated fat and 95 or fewer milligrams of cholesterol per serving
Extra lean	5 or fewer grams of fat, 2 or fewer grams of saturated fat and 95 or fewer milligrams of cholesterol per serving
High	20 percent or more of the Percent Daily Value for a nutrient such as a vitamin, mineral or fiber; "excellent source of" and "rich in" may also be used
Good source	10 percent to 19 percent of the Percent Daily Value for a nutrient
More	10 percent or more of the Percent Daily Value for a nutrient; "enriched," "fortified" and "added" may also be used
Healthy	Low in fat and saturated fat, 480 or fewer milligrams of sodium and at least 10 percent of the Percent Daily Value of vitamin A, vitamin C, calcium, iron, protein and fiber per serving

Notes

1. All information for the health benefits section for each food group came from: U.S. Department of Health and Human Services and U.S. Department of Agriculture, *Dietary Guidelines for Americans, 2005, 6th edition*, Washington, DC: U.S. Government Printing Office, January 2005.
2. USFDA/CFSAN. *How to Understand and Use the Nutrition Facts Label*, November 2004. http://www.cfsan.fda.gov/~dms/foodlab.html (accessed November 2007).
3. American Heart Association. *Know Your Fats*. September 5, 2007. http://www.americanheart.org/presenter.jhtml?identifier=532 (accessed November 2007).
4. USFDA/CFSAN. *Questions and Answers About Trans Fat Nutrition Labeling*, January 1, 2006. http://www.cfsan.fda.gov/~dms/qatrans2.html (accessed November 2007).
5. Institute of Medicine (U.S.) Panel on Dietary Reference Intakes for Electrolytes and Water. Dietary reference intakes for water, potassium, sodium, chloride, and sulfate / Panel on Dietary Reference Intakes for Electrolytes and Water, Standing Committee on the Scientific Evaluation of Dietary Reference Intakes, Food and Nutrition Board. 2005. The National Academies Press. http://www.nap.edu (accessed November 2007).

a cure for
portion distortion

Q*uality* and *quantity* are both important principles when it comes to lasting weight loss and adopting healthy eating habits for life. Choosing *quality* foods that are nutrient dense (as opposed to calorie dense) help us get the proper nutrients our body needs for maintenance and health, and *quality* foods tend to deliver these nutrients with a much cheaper caloric price tag. However, some foods rich in nutrients can still provide a lot of calories, such as avocados and nuts. Does this mean you shouldn't eat them? Are they banned from your repertoire of foods forever? Absolutely not! Balancing *quality* foods in the *appropriate quantities* is the solution!

DINING IN AMERICA—DIAL 911!

If you even casually observe the portions provided at most restaurants today, you can easily see that the portions do not even come close to lining up with suggested serving sizes. In fact, they are usually double or triple in size! Today, bagels look like mini-life-rafts; "super-sizing" is practically a household term; and you may even get your wallet slapped (by way of a "splitting charge") if you make the remarkably reasonable and wise decision to share your favorite restaurant's bowl-the-size-of-a-birdbath of spaghetti with your spouse or a friend.

Times have definitely changed when it comes to dining in America. For example, in 1960, a bagel weighed 3 ounces and provided about 140 calories. Today, the average bagel weighs 6 ounces—an amount that satisfies most adults' grain servings for an entire day—and provides around 350 calories! Twenty years ago, a 2.4-ounce (now deemed "small") serving of French fries provided 210 calories; but today the popular 6.9-ounce serving ("large") is going to cost you a lot more—610 calories![1]

All signs point to this bottom line: Don't expect sensible portions to be handed to you on a moderately sized silver platter (even plates have increased in size over the years)! However, many simple and commonsense tools exist to assist you in escaping the ever-present lure of portion distortion! First, take a closer look at portions versus servings. Believe it or not, the terms are not synonymous.

PORTIONS VERSUS SERVINGS

It is very important to understand the difference between a portion and a serving. One self-determined portion may not equal one standardized serving. You (or the person plating your food) determine how big or small your portions are. Whether you are eating in a restaurant or plating dinner in your own kitchen, a portion size is how much food you put on your plate and *choose* to eat. The portion sizes you are used to eating may be equal to two or three standard servings.

The U.S. government, specifically the FDA, determines the size of one serving of a particular food. A serving size is the amount of food listed on the product's Nutrition Facts Panel and is not necessarily the recommended amount to eat. Sometimes, the typical portion size and serving size for a product match; sometimes they do not. For example, a 1-ounce slice of bread is considered a serving for the grains group. However, a typical portion of bread for a sandwich includes two slices. This is perfectly appropriate—you just need to be aware that the bread for your sandwich has fulfilled two of your daily suggested servings for the grains group.

Portion: The amount of food you choose to eat for a meal or snack—the size is up to you. A portion should be appropriately sized to provide adequate servings for one or more food groups, according to your calorie range, but not provide servings in excess of the recommended amounts.

Serving: A standard amount of food or drink, such as 1 slice of bread or 1 cup of milk, as determined by the U.S. government.

PORTION REALITY CHECK

So how do you know if your portions are too big? And how can you control them? First, figure out how many calories you need in order to lose weight slowly (no more than two pounds a week) or to maintain your ideal body weight.

Second, refer to MyPyramid table to see how many servings from each food group are recommended for your calorie range. For example, if you are aiming for a daily caloric intake of 1,600 calories, your day's total meals should include the following:

- $1^1/_2$ to 2 cups of mostly fruit, some juice
- 2 to $2^1/_2$ cups of a variety of veggies
- 5 to 6 ounce equivalents of grains (at least half should be whole)

- 5 to 5$^1/_2$ ounce equivalents of lean meat, beans, nuts and seeds
- 3 cups of skim or low-fat milk or milk products
- 4 to 5 teaspoons of healthy oils (including oils in certain foods)

Now, use the tools available to you on a daily basis to help remind yourself how much you really need to eat.

Read Food Labels

Ingredients lists are on almost every food container in your kitchen. They are even available at most restaurants! Learn how much of something actually makes up one serving. All you have to do is look at the serving size listed on the Nutrition Facts Panel. How many ounces are in one serving of your favorite snack crackers? How many cups of yogurt are provided in the container in your refrigerator? Just take a few moments to glance at the back of the containers—it's a simple and effective way to monitor how much food and drink you're consuming. (*Note:* Low-fat items count toward daily calories and nutrients, too, so don't write them off as freebies.)

Measure to Discover

Take 30 minutes and discover what $^1/_2$ cup of rice, 2 tablespoons of butter or 1 cup of vegetables looks like. You don't have to measure and count everything you eat for the rest of your life; just do it long enough to discover how much you're *actually* eating compared to how much you *should* be eating. For example, do you know how much room a 3-ounce portion of chicken takes up on your plate? Try it and find out! You may be surprised at how much you've been accustomed to eating for breakfast, lunch and dinner. Learn to visualize portions! Once you familiarize yourself with what actual appropriate servings for various foods look like, you will grow increasingly more skilled at eyeballing portions in the future.

Use Visual Cues

When you don't have a scale or measuring cup on hand, you still have no excuse not to estimate portion sizes. You have a fist or various household items to help guide you in estimating proper portion sizes. Check out the table on page 159 for easy visual clues to use to maintain portion control wherever you are—at home or away.

Other Remedies for Portion Distortion

Remember number 10 on the Nutrition Top 10 list: *Practice mindfulness.* Always be aware of what you are eating and drinking. Mental awareness goes a long way toward managing your portions. Here are more tips to assist you in curing portion distortion:

- Use your Live It Tracker, and practice keeping track of your portions. Write down when, what, how much, where and why you eat. This will help you become more aware of the amount of food you are eating and the times you tend to eat too much.

- Avoid eating packaged food without looking at the NFP first. Measure out an appropriate portion by referring to the recommended serving size listed on the label.

- Turn off the TV at meal or snack times. This will increase your mindfulness of what you are eating.

- Relish the home advantage—home cooking, that is! Take control of what you ingest, and enjoy preparing something healthy that does not contain any mystery ingredients.

- Don't feel pressured to clean your plate. Savor each bite, eat slowly, listen to your hunger cues, and remove yourself from food once the meal is over—don't linger at the table!

- Freeze what's left over when you cook a large meal (such as soup or a casserole) so that you won't be tempted to finish it off after you've already eaten your dinner.

- Try using a smaller plate. Studies show that people who eat on a larger plate tend to fill their plate with more food and eat it all; yet, the quantity of food on a smaller plate is just as satisfying.

- Split meals with a companion at restaurants—it's worth the extra money if there is a charge to split the food. Or ask for a to-go box as soon as you get your meal, and pack up half for tomorrow so that you can truly enjoy only what you need for today. Some restaurants will do this for you—just ask!

- Don't be bullied! Even the most well-intentioned waitpersons can pressure customers to order more than they need. Exercise your rights as a consumer, and order what you know is right for you—and no more.

WEBSITES OF INTEREST

Food Labeling and Nutrition: www.cfsan.fda.gov/label.html

The New American Plate: www.aicr.org/site/PageServer?pagename=pub_nap_index_21

Portion Distortion Interactive Quiz: hp2010.nhlbihin.net/portion/

FOOD AND AMOUNT	VISUAL CUE
Grains Group	
1-ounce bread slice	Computer disk
1 cup ready-to-eat cereal (flakes)	Baseball, clenched fist
$1/2$ cup cooked cereal, rice, pasta	Tennis ball, cupcake wrapper (full)
1 pancake	Compact disc
1 piece cornbread	Bar of soap
1 ounce pretzels, $1/3$ cup popcorn	Rounded handful
Vegetable Group	
$1/2$ cup cooked vegetables	Rounded handful, ice cream scoop, lightbulb
1 cup raw leafy greens, 1 baked potato, $1/2$ cup cooked dry beans	Baseball, clenched fist, computer mouse
Fruit Group	
1 medium piece of fruit	Baseball
$1/2$ cup chopped, cooked or canned fruit	Rounded handful, ice cream scoop, lightbulb
$1/4$ cup dried fruit or raisins	Large egg, golf ball
Milk Group	
1 cup milk or yogurt	Baseball, small milk carton
$1/2$ cup ice cream	Half of a baseball
$1 1/2$ ounces natural cheese	two 9-volt batteries or 4 dice
Meat and Beans Group	
2 tablespoons or 1 ounce peanut butter	Ping-Pong ball or roll of film
3 ounces meat or poultry	Deck of cards
3 ounces fish	Checkbook
1 ounce nuts	Small handful
Oils	
1 teaspoon butter or margarine	Fingertip, 1 dice
2 tablespoons salad dressing	Ping-Pong ball

Note

1. "Portion Distortion—Do You Know How Food Portions Have Changed in 20 Years?" National Heart, Lung, and Blood Institute. http://hp2010.nhlbihin.net/portion/index.htm (accessed February 2008).

eating healthy
when eating out!

National survey data show a significant trend in the dining styles of most Americans over the past few decades: Eating away from home is increasing in popularity. From 1999 to 2000, more Americans ate out and ate out more frequently than in 1987 or 1992. Specifically, the odds of eating out at least one or more meals per day and three or more meals per week was 40 percent higher in 1999-2000 relative to 1987.[1] Whether the reason is time, convenience, variety or value, Americans waste no time pulling into the local drive-thru or diner—even for breakfast.

Unfortunately, a higher frequency of eating out has been shown to be associated with adverse nutritional consequences. Despite the fact that many consumers agree that they are ultimately responsible for making sensible food choices away from home, French fries continue to trump green salads as a side dish.

Believe it or not, you can dine out without blowing it; you just need to know how. The keys to success are having a plan for healthy eating, sticking with it and exercising your rights as a consumer by asking for exactly what you want!

YOUR RIGHT TO EAT HEALTHY!

When you breeze through the doors of your favorite restaurant, you are not entering a world where calories do not count and fat does not exist. Rather, calories can add up even more quickly, and fat is usually lurking in every corner. It is your responsibility to overcome the temptation to let ignorance be your bliss. (And it's also your choice to remind yourself that the bliss will come to a screeching halt the next morning when you try to fasten your pants!)

Some restaurants do a great job of informing their patrons about the nutritional content of menu items, but most won't unless you ask. The good news is that if they want your business, they will most certainly oblige! So remind yourself that you are paying not only for the experience of the meal but also for the meal itself. Get what you paid for, namely, a healthy and delicious product! Don't think that you're being picky; you're being *proactive*. Ask questions and act accordingly—it's perfectly polite!

Ask if the restaurant will do the following:

- Serve your salad dressing and other condiments on the side.
- Substitute fresh salad greens or grilled veggies for fried sides.
- Serve margarine rather than butter.
- Serve fat-free or low-fat milk rather than whole milk or cream.
- Accommodate special requests for menu items.
- Bring a side of lemon or lime slices to flavor your water.
- Use whole-wheat bread or pasta.
- Use less oil when cooking.
- Hold the salt, or use salt-free seasoning instead.
- Trim visible fat from poultry or meat.
- Leave off the sauce or substitute it with a different, lower-calorie kind.
- Split the entrée ahead of time, and bring it on two separate plates.

Choose what is better (and still very delicious!).

- Remember number 6 on the Nutrition Top 10, and choose better beverages! Don't waste your calories on sugar-filled beverages with no nutritional value! Opt for water (add some lemon or lime if you wish), unsweetened tea that you can sweeten yourself, fat-free or low-fat milk, or (occasionally) diet drinks.
- Start off with a salad to help you control hunger and feel satisfied sooner. It's also an easy way to get your veggies!
- Order pasta dishes with tomato-based sauces (such as marinara) more often than cream-based sauces (like Alfredo sauce). Try to stick to items without creamy sauces or gravies.
- Add little or no butter to your food. If you get out of the habit of adding butter, you'll realize that you don't miss anything but the extra calories!
- Bypass the all-you-can-eat buffets, and order an item from the menu instead.
- If chips or bread are being served as complimentary appetizers, ask the waiter to bring only one basket, and spare yourself extra temptation.
- Most often choose fruit-based desserts. Split the rich ones with your companions.

- Big portions are a problem when eating out. Almost any restaurant meal can be a good choice if you don't eat all of it. Shift your membership from the clean-plate club to the *lean*-plate club; stop when you've had enough, and leave or pack up the rest. The key to controlling portions is to have a plan before you order.

USE CLUES TO COMPARE

Menus are full of food clues, if you know what to look for. Start choosing more items prepared using healthier methods. Here are lists of terms you'll read on menus. Make a note of the terms that describe foods that would be best for you to choose.

Choose Most Often	Choose Seldom
Baked	Deep fried
Broiled	Pan fried
Roasted	Sautéed (using a lot of butter or oil)
Braised	Prime
Poached	Casserole
Steamed	Breaded
Stir-fried	Alfredo or cream sauce
Grilled	
Sautéed (with broth, cooking spray or minimal oil)	
Tomato sauce	

TAKE A TASTE ADVENTURE

Maintaining variety in your diet is not only essential for nutrition, but it also makes eating fun and exciting! Experiencing new cuisines from around the world is a wonderful way to gain respect for other cultures as well as tickle your taste buds with fresh and delicious new foods. Many ethnic cuisines offer lots of low-fat, low-calorie choices. Here's a sample of healthy food choices and terms to look for when making your selection:

Asian	Italian	Mexican
Jum (poached)	Red sauces (marinara, pomodoro)	Grilled chicken fajitas
Kow (roasted)	Primavera (no cream)	Black beans
Shu (barbecued)	Piccata (lemon)	Charo beans
Steamed dumplings (rice, chicken or shrimp)	Sun-dried tomatoes	Salsa or picante
Dishes without MSG	Crushed tomatoes	Pico de gallo
	Lightly sautéed	Soft corn tortillas
	Whole-wheat pizza crust	

BETTER CHOICES AT ANY MEAL

A Healthy Start

- Choose toast, a small (or half) bagel or English muffin with a small amount of margarine or low-fat cream cheese and jam or jelly. Add nonfat milk and fruit or fruit juice to balance out your meal.

- Cold or hot cereals with nonfat milk are a great start to any day. Top the cereal with fresh or dried fruit for added nutrition. Choose wholesome cereals with little or no added sugar and 3 or more grams of fiber.

- Limit eggs (two or three each week), bacon, sausage, fried potatoes, biscuits, croissants and sweet rolls. Muffins can be high in calories and fat and sugar, so be sure to read labels or ask for the nutrition facts.

Midday Munching

- Broth-based soups and fresh salads with dressing on the side make a great noontime choice. Watch out for cream-based soups and potato, macaroni, tuna or chicken salads that are usually made with full-fat mayonnaise. Ask if the chef can provide lighter versions of those items.

- Choose sandwiches with grilled chicken, lean roast beef, turkey or ham. Some deli-style sandwiches pack on the meat; ask for more vegetables instead. Order mustard or low-fat spreads instead of mayonnaise.

- Limit French fries, onion rings and chips. Ask that they be left off your plate, or substitute a baked potato, fruit or vegetables. Burgers and hot dogs are okay occasionally, but avoid the deluxe versions.

A Night Out

- Choose baked, broiled or grilled chicken (without the skin), fish or small portions of lean meats. Limit fried and prime cuts of meat and heavy sauces.

- Pastas with tomato-based sauces and fresh vegetables are good choices. Limit cream- or cheese-based sauces. When you do order them, ask that they be served on the side.

- Start your meal with a fresh salad and broth-based soup to help control your appetite. Better yet, when you know that you will be dining out, eat a piece of fruit or drink a glass of nonfat milk before you go.

Satisfy Your Sweet Tooth

- First ask yourself if you're really hungry. If you're not, have dessert at another time. If you are hungry, the best choices include fresh fruit, sorbet, frozen yogurt, sherbet or angel food cake with a fruit topping.

- Desserts aren't always off limits—just keep your overall goals in mind. If you know ahead of time that you will order dessert, plan to split your favorite treat with a companion. Another option is to eat slowly and to eat only a few bites while savoring each one!

PREPARE TO ENJOY!

When eating out with family and friends, tell them in advance that you plan to eat healthy. Order what you know is best for you, and don't allow yourself to be tempted by others (including the waitstaff!). Also, if you know that a meal will be high in calories and fat, choose more healthy foods during the rest of the day and be more physically active.

In the following table, list the restaurants where you dine most often. Next, list the foods that you usually order. What foods would be better choices?

Restaurant	Usual Choices (Be specific)	Better Choices

Reward yourself when you make good choices.

Note

1. A. K. Kant and B. I. Graubard, "Eating Out in America, 1987-2000: Trends and Nutritional Correlates," *Preventive Medicine*, vol. 38 (2004), pp. 243-249.

modifying recipes

Low-fat cookbooks fill bookstore and library shelves. Perhaps you even have a collection of favorite low-fat—or even regular—cookbooks on your bookshelf. If you like to cook and learn new recipes, that's great. But for most of us, learning to prepare all new recipes is not realistic.

Fortunately, you don't have to buy a new cookbook or learn all new recipes to eat healthy and lose weight. You can make almost any recipe healthier with a few simple changes. Use the following tips to help turn your recipes into healthier alternatives. (*Note:* Many modern cookbooks include substitution lists in the appendix, so check your cookbooks for such lists.)

START WITH THE BASICS

- Start by looking at ways to cut calories, fat, sugar and sodium. Often you can achieve this by simply choosing the lighter options of various products (in other words, choose light sour cream, low-sodium soups, extra-lean ground beef, and so forth).

- Increase the nutritional value of your recipes by adding or substituting more healthful foods (whole grains, vegetables, legumes and fruits) for less healthful foods (high-fat meats and refined grains).

- Make changes gradually to learn what works best. Changing ingredients can affect taste, texture and appearance, so you may have to do some experimenting.

- For that special occasion when you don't want to change your favorite recipe, just serve smaller portions.

USE SUBSTITUTIONS FOR HEALTHY COOKING AND BAKING

ITEM	SUBSTITUTION
Bacon or sausage	Lean turkey bacon, Canadian bacon
Beef	Chicken or turkey without skin
Ground beef	Lean or extra-lean ground turkey breast
1 cup butter, margarine or oil for baking (up to half can be substituted)	$^1/_2$ cup apple butter or applesauce, pureed prunes or plums
Butter, margarine, or vegetable oil for sautéing	Cooking spray, low-fat or nonfat chicken broth, or a small amount of olive oil
Cake (pound, chocolate or yellow)	Angel food cake, white cake, gingerbread
1 cup cream cheese	$^1/_2$ cup ricotta cheese pureed with 1/2 cup fat-free cream cheese, Neufchatel or "light" cream cheese
1 cup chocolate chips	$^1/_4$ to $^1/_2$ cup mini-chocolate chips
1 cup heavy cream	1 cup evaporated fat-free milk
1 cup sour cream	1 cup plain nonfat yogurt, 1 cup 1 percent cottage cheese plus 2 teaspoons lemon juice, or low-fat varieties of sour cream
Whipping cream	Imitation whipped cream made with skim milk
1 egg	2 egg whites or $^1/_4$ cup egg substitute _1 Med egg_
Ice cream	Sorbet, sherbet, low-fat soy ice cream, low-fat frozen yogurt
1 cup regular mayonnaise	1 cup reduced-fat or light mayonnaise
Meat	Tofu, beans, lentils or other vegetables
1 cup whole milk	1 cup skim, $^1/_2$ percent or 1 percent milk
Nuts	Grapenuts
Oil and vinegar dressing with 3 parts oil to 1 part vinegar	1 part olive oil plus 1 part flavored vinegar (balsamic) plus 1 part orange juice
Pastry dough/pie crust	Graham-cracker crust
Ramen noodles	Rice or noodles
Salt (for cooking, not baking)	Herbs, spices, salt-free seasoning blends
1 cup sugar	$^3/_4$ cup sugar (this works with most everything except yeast breads)
Tortilla chips (fried)	Homemade baked tortillas (divide into four, baste with a little olive oil and salt, and bake)
Unsweetened baking chocolate (1 oz.)	3 tablespoons unsweetened cocoa powder plus 1 tablespoon canola oil, peanut oil or margarine appropriate for baking

CUT THE FAT

■ Broil, grill, roast or bake instead of frying meat, poultry and fish. Use a rack or pans designed to catch drippings so that your meat won't cook in its own fat. Use lean meats trimmed of visible fat and skin.

■ Baste, broil and stir-fry using small amounts of oil, broth, water or fruit juice. Use vegetable-oil spray and nonstick pots and pans instead of oils and butter.

- Limit meat portions in your recipes to 3 ounces or less per serving. Make up for the reduced meat by adding more grains (rice or pasta), vegetables or legumes.

- Use meat alternatives—beans, lentils, peas or soy products—in recipes that call for meat.

- Drain fat from meat during or after cooking. Rinse cooked ground meat with hot water to remove much of the fat.

- Refrigerate soups and stews before serving. Remove the layer of fat that forms at the top and hardens after cooling.

- In recipes calling for eggs, use cholesterol-free egg substitutes, or substitute two egg whites for every whole egg.

- To cut the fat in a recipe by one-third to one-half, use vegetable oils instead of butter or shortening, and use low-fat dairy products.

- In recipes calling for cheese, use one-third to one-half of what the recipe calls for. Use low-fat cheese with 3 to 5 grams of fat per 1-ounce serving.

- Use nonfat sour cream or make your own by mixing $1/2$ cup low-fat yogurt and $1/2$ cup low-fat cottage cheese. Flavor with lemon juice and your favorite herbs and spices.

- Replace some of the fat in baked goods with fruit purées (such as prune, apple-sauce or banana) or nonfat dairy products (such as nonfat yogurt). Use $1/2$ cup of puréed fruit in place of 1 cup of butter, shortening or oil. Don't get rid of all the fat. You may need to add 1 to 2 tablespoons of fat back into the recipe to achieve the best results.

- Use low-fat or nonfat cream cheese, sour cream, yogurt, mayonnaise and salad dressing instead of the full-fat versions.

CUT THE SUGAR

- Try using one-fourth to one-third less sugar than what the recipe calls for.

- Substitute artificial sweeteners when appropriate. Keep in mind, though, that this will not work in many baked goods. Aspartame (used in NutraSweet and in Equal artificial sweeteners) cannot be used in cooking—it loses its sweetness when heated. Splenda artificial sweetener, however, can be used in cooking and baking.

- Learn to make special treats with fruits, such as fruit and yogurt smoothies, fruit pops, frozen bananas and trail mix.

- Experiment using fruit juice concentrates instead of sugar. If you do this though, you'll need to reduce the amount of overall liquid ingredients.

- Serve smaller portions of your favorite recipes.

CUT THE SODIUM

- Add flavor to vegetables, meats, poultry and fish by using herbs and spices instead of salt or high-sodium seasonings or sauces.

- Choose low-sodium versions of soups, broths and sauces.

- Eliminate or cut the salt in half for most of your recipes. Many seasoning packets in easy-to-fix meals (for example, macaroni and cheese) are high in sodium. Use one-half or less of the packet, or substitute your own seasonings.

- Rinse canned vegetables with water to wash away extra sodium.

ADD FIBER, VITAMINS AND MINERALS

- Increase fiber by substituting whole-wheat flour, oats or cornmeal for some of the flour in recipes. Substitute with whole-wheat flour one-half of white flour in a recipe, or substitute one-third of white flour with oats.

- Add puréed fruits or vegetables in place of some of the water in recipes.

- Keep the peels on fruits and vegetables such as potatoes, carrots and apples.

- Add extra vegetables or grains such as rice, pasta or legumes to soups, sauces, salads and casseroles.

- Top a baked potato with steamed, fresh or stir-fried vegetables.

GLOSSARY OF HERBS AND SPICES

Herbs are the aromatic leaves of plants without woody stems that grow in temperate zones. *Spices* are seasonings obtained from the bark, buds, fruit or flower parts, roots, seeds or stems of various aromatic plants and trees. Both should be stored in airtight glass jars in a cool, dark place for no more than six months.

Allspice: Dark-brown, pea-size berries from the evergreen pimento tree. Flavor is pungent, sweet mixture of cinnamon, clove and nutmeg flavors. Use in breads, cakes, cookies and fruit sauces.

Basil: Most varieties are green leaves; member of the mint family. Flavor is sweet, clovelike and pungent. Use with chicken, eggs, fish, pasta and tomatoes and in Italian and Mediterranean recipes.

Bay Leaf: Leaves from the evergreen bay laurel tree; also called bay laurel or laurel leaf. Flavor is woodsy and pungent. Use for meats, pickling, sauces, soups, stews and vegetables.

Chili Powder: Seasoning blend made from ground dried chilies, coriander, cumin, garlic, oregano and other herbs and spices. Flavor is mild to hot. Use in chili, eggs, cheese, soups and stews.

Cilantro: Bright-green stems and leaves from the coriander plant; also called coriander and Chinese parsley. Flavor is pungent and spicy. Use with fish, rice, salsas and salads and in Italian, Latin American and Mexican recipes.

Cinnamon: Bark from the Ceylon (buff colored) or Cassia tree (dark reddish brown). Flavor is aromatic, pungent and sweet. Cinnamon sticks are added to dishes during the cooking process for flavor but are not meant to be eaten. Use in cakes, cookies, hot drinks, pies and vegetables (carrots, winter squash, sweet potatoes).

Cloves: Reddish-brown, nail-shaped buds from the tropical evergreen clove tree. Flavor is aromatic, pungent and sweet. Cloves should be used with care as the flavor can become overpowering. Use for baked beans, fruit pies, ham, pickling, sauces, spice cakes and cookies.

Cumin: Dried fruit from a plant in the parsley family. Flavor is slightly bitter, pungent, nutty and hot. Use in chili and curry-powder blends, fish, lamb, pickling and sausages and in Middle Eastern, Asian and Mediterranean recipes.

Dill Seed (spice): Dried seed from the dill plant. Flavor is tangy. Use in meats, salads, sauces and vegetables.

Dill Weed (herb): Feathery green leaves from the dill plant. Flavor is pungent and tangy. Use for breads, fish, pickling, salads, sauces and vegetables.

Fennel Seeds: Oval, greenish-brown seeds from the fennel plant. Flavor is aromatic and slightly like licorice. Use for breads, fish, sauces, sausage, soups and salad dressings and in Italian recipes.

Ginger: Gnarled and bumpy root from the ginger plant. Flavor is peppery, slightly sweet with a pungent and spicy aroma. Use for cakes, cookies and marinades and in Chinese, Jamaican and German recipes. Don't substitute dry ginger powder for recipes specifying fresh ginger.

Marjoram: Oval, inch-long pale-green leaves; member of the mint/oregano family. Flavor is aromatic and slightly bitter. Use for fish, meat, poultry, sausages, stuffings and vegetables.

Mint: Peppermint and spearmint are two of the most popular kinds of the 25 or more varieties that exist. Flavor is strong and sweet, with a cool aftertaste. Use in beverages, desserts, lamb, sauces and soups.

Nutmeg: Gray-brown oval seeds from the nutmeg tree. (Mace is the spice obtained from the membrane of the seeds.) Flavor is nutty, warm, spicy and sweet. Use in beverages, cakes, cookies, sauces and sweet potatoes.

Oregano: Member of the mint family, related to marjoram and thyme. Flavor is strong and aromatic, with a pungent marjoram flavor. Use for fish, meat, poultry and tomatoes and in Greek, Italian and Mexican recipes.

Paprika: Dried red peppers ground into a powder. Flavor is slightly bitter, ranging from sweet to hot. Use for dips, fish, poultry, salads (potato and egg) and soups and in goulash.

Parsley: Curly leaf and Italian (flat-leaf) parsley are only two of the more popular varieties that exist. Flavor is slightly peppery. Use sprigs as garnish and in herb mixtures, sauces, soups and stews.

Rosemary: Silver-green, needle-shaped leaves; member of the mint family. Flavor is sweet with hints of lemon and pine. Use in casseroles, fish, fruit salads, lamb, soups and stuffings.

Sage: Narrow, oval gray-green leaves. Flavor is musty, minty and slightly bitter. Use in chicken, duck, goose, pork, sausages and stuffings.

Thyme: Garden thyme (most common) is a bush with gray-green leaves; member of the mint family. The flavor is pungent, minty and tealike. Use for fish, meats, poultry, soups and vegetables (eggplants, mushrooms, potatoes and summer squash).

SAMPLE RECIPE MAKEOVERS

Lasagna

Original Recipe	Modified Recipe
1 box lasagna noodles	1 box whole-wheat lasagna noodles
1 pound ground beef	1 pound 90-95% lean ground beef or lean/extra lean turkey
$1/2$ cup chopped onion	$1/2$ cup chopped onion
8 ounces mushrooms (optional)	8 ounces mushrooms (optional)
1 16-ounce jar spaghetti sauce	1 16-ounce jar spaghetti sauce with no added fat and least amount added sugar
1 teaspoon garlic powder	1 to 2 cloves garlic
$1/2$ teaspoon salt	$1/2$ teaspoon salt
1 teaspoon dried oregano	1 teaspoon dried oregano
$1/2$ teaspoon dried basil	$1/2$ teaspoon dried basil
1 $1/2$ cups ricotta cheese	1 $1/2$ cups part-skim ricotta cheese
2 cups shredded Monterey Jack cheese	2 cups shredded reduced-fat Monterey Jack cheese
$3/4$ cup grated Parmesan cheese	$3/4$ cup grated reduced-fat Parmesan cheese

Cook lasagna noodles according to package directions, drain and set aside. In a large skillet brown beef, onion and mushrooms. Stir in spaghetti sauce, garlic powder, salt, oregano, and basil into meat. In a 2-quart buttered baking dish (11" x 7" x 2"), layer pasta, cheeses and meat sauce. Repeat layers until finished. Bake lasagna for 30 minutes or until thoroughly heated and bubbly. Let stand 8-10 minutes before cutting and serving. Serves 6 to 8.

Whole-wheat noodles may need a few extra minutes to soften. Use little or no added oil to grease the pan. Be sure to drain the fat from the meat after you brown it. Stir in spaghetti sauce, garlic powder, salt, oregano, and basil into meat. In a 2-quart buttered baking dish (11" x 7" x 2"), layer pasta, cheeses and meat sauce. Repeat layers until finished. Bake lasagna for 30 minutes or until thoroughly heated and bubbly. Let stand 8-10 minutes before cutting and serving. Serves 6 to 8.

Selected Values per serving:

Calories: 549	Total Fat: 33 g
Fiber: 3 g	Cholesterol: 96 mg
Sodium: 749 mg	

Selected Values per serving:

Calories: 399 (less than original!)	Total Fat: 18 g (less!)
Fiber: 6 g (more!)	Cholesterol: 83 mg (less!)
Sodium: 691 mg (less!)	

Coffee Cake

Original Recipe

1 $1/2$ cups flour

$3/4$ cup sugar

1 egg

$1/2$ cup milk

$1/4$ cup shortening

2 teaspoons baking powder

$1/2$ teaspoon salt

Topping:

$1/2$ cup brown sugar

2 teaspoons flour

2 teaspoons cinnamon

2 tablespoons butter

Preheat oven to 350°F and grease an 8" or 9" cake pan. Combine sugar, shortening and egg. Stir in milk. Combine flour, baking powder and salt. Gradually add this to the wet ingredients and mix until smooth. Pour half of the batter into the greased cake pan and set aside as you prepare the topping. For the topping, soften the butter and mix in the brown sugar, flour and cinnamon. Spoon half of the topping over the first layer and spoon on the rest of the topping. Bake 25-30 minutes.

Selected Values per serving:

Calories: 156

Saturated fat: 1.7 g

Fiber: 0.5 g

Total fat: 5.0 g

Cholesterol: 16 mg

Sodium: 159 mg

Modified Recipe

$3/4$ cup all-purpose flour and $1/2$ cup whole-wheat flour

$1/2$ cup sugar

1 beaten egg

$1/4$ cup skim milk, rice milk or soy milk

$2/3$ cup plain fat-free yogurt and 2 tablespoons canola oil

$3/4$ teaspoon baking powder and $1/4$ teaspoon baking soda

$1/4$ teaspoon salt

$1/4$ teaspoon ground nutmeg

$1/2$ teaspoon vanilla

Topping:

1 medium mango, peeled, seeded, and finely chopped (about 1 cup)

1 tablespoon all-purpose flour

2 tablespoons shredded coconut

Preheat oven to 350°F and lightly spray 8" x 8" square pan with cooking spray and then dust with flour. Set aside. Combine both flours, sugar, baking powder, baking soda, salt and nutmeg. Set aside. Combine egg, yogurt, milk, oil and vanilla. Add the egg mixture all at once to the flour mixture. Stir until just moistened (batter may be slightly lumpy). Toss the mango with 1 tablespoon of flour and gently fold into batter. Spread batter into prepared pan. Sprinkle coconut over batter and bake for 30-35 minutes.

Selected Values per serving:

Calories: 97 (less than original!)

Saturated fat: 0.5 g (less!)

Fiber: 1.0 g (more!)

Total fat: 2.5 g (less!)

Cholesterol: 12 mg (less!)

Sodium: 114 mg (less!)

After reviewing the suggested modifications for various ingredients, choose a few recipes for which you're willing to make changes. List them below, along with the ingredients and healthy substitutions.

Recipe/Food	Preparation/Ingredients	Healthy Change

Recipe/Food   Preparation/Ingredients   Healthy Change

_____

Recipe/Food   Preparation/Ingredients   Healthy Change

_____

Recipe/Food   Preparation/Ingredients   Healthy Change

_____

live it the vegetarian way!

Most experts now agree that a well-planned vegetarian eating program can supply all the nutrients your body needs for good health. In fact, research shows that eating the vegetarian way can reduce the risk for many health problems, such as coronary heart disease, high blood pressure, diabetes and some forms of cancer. Of course, any eating plan that's well balanced and includes a variety of foods can lower your risk for disease and improve your overall health and quality of life.

Several different vegetarian eating plans exist. The following is a list of the most common variations:

- *Vegans* are strict vegetarians who eat only plant foods such as fruits, vegetables, legumes (dried beans and peas), grains, seeds and nuts.
- *Lacto-vegetarians* include cheese and other dairy products in their diet.
- *Lacto-ovo vegetarians* include both eggs and dairy products.
- *Semi-vegetarians* exclude red meat but occasionally include poultry and fish.

NUTRIENTS TO FOCUS ON

The key in a vegetarian food plan is to consume a variety of foods in appropriate amounts in order to meet your daily caloric and nutrient needs. Specifically, nutrients that vegetarians need to focus on include protein, iron, calcium, zinc and vitamin B_{12}.

Protein

Protein has many important functions in the body and is essential for growth and maintenance. Protein needs can easily be met by eating a variety of plant-based foods such as beans, nuts, nut butters, peas and soy products (tofu, tempeh and veggie burgers). Milk products and eggs are also good protein sources for lacto-ovo vegetarians.

Iron

Iron carries oxygen to various tissues through the blood. Iron sources for vegetarians include iron-fortified cereals, spinach, kidney beans, black-eyed peas, lentils, turnip greens, molasses, whole-wheat breads, peas and some dried fruits.

Calcium

Calcium is essential for the health of your bones and teeth. Vegetarian sources of calcium include fortified cereals, soy products, calcium-fortified orange juice and some dark-green leafy vegetables such as collard greens, turnip greens, bok choy and mustard greens. Milk and other dairy products are excellent sources of calcium for lacto-vegetarians.

Zinc

Zinc is a necessary element for many biochemical reactions as well as for proper immune-system function. Vegetarian sources of zinc include many types of beans, zinc-fortified cereals, wheat germ and pumpkin seeds. Milk and other dairy products are also appropriate sources of zinc for lacto-vegetarians.

Vitamin B_{12}

Vitamin B_{12} is found mostly in animal products but also in some fortified foods such as milk and other dairy products, eggs, fortified cereals, soy-based beverages, veggie burgers and nutritional yeast.

A HEALTHY VEGETARIAN FOOD PLAN

A properly planned vegetarian diet includes adequate amounts of protein, calories, vitamins and minerals and is low in saturated fat, total fat and cholesterol. Furthermore, a variety of foods—including whole grains, vegetables, fruits, legumes, nuts, seeds and low-fat dairy products and eggs, if desired—should contribute to a balanced vegetarian diet. But remember, the same principles of healthy eating that apply to non-vegetarian diets also apply to vegetarian diets: quality and quantity are key!

Build meals around protein sources that are naturally low in fat, such as beans, lentils and rice. Don't overload meals with high-fat cheeses to replace meat. (*Note:* Eating vegetarian doesn't necessarily mean eating low-fat. Many meat alternatives such as dairy can be higher in fat and calories than meat.)

Don't skimp on protein! Legumes, nuts, seeds, peanut butter, eggs and tofu are all excellent sources of vegetarian protein. Consider the following foods (all represent one serving per food group):

- 1 cup milk, soy milk or other dairy product (products fortified with calcium, vitamin D and vitamin B_{12})

- $1/4$ cup cooked dry or canned beans or peas
- 2 tablespoons hummus
- 1 egg
- 2 tablespoons nuts or seeds
- $1/4$ cup tofu, soy cheese or tempeh
- 1 tablespoon peanut or other nut butters

A NOTE ABOUT SOY

Animal proteins are considered complete proteins because they supply all the essential amino acids your body needs, while most plant-based proteins come up short in one or two of these acids. However, soy-protein products can be good substitutes for animal products because, unlike some other beans, soy offers a complete protein profile. In other words, soybeans contain all the amino acids essential to human nutrition, which must be supplied in the diet because they cannot be synthesized by the human body.

TIPS FOR VEGETARIANS

- Many dishes that usually contain meat or poultry can be made vegetarian by substituting the meat or poultry with one of many vegetarian options (vegetables, legumes, soy products, yogurt and various grains). These include pasta primavera, marinara or pesto sauce with vegetables; veggie pizza; vegetable lasagna; tofu-veggie stir-fry with brown rice; vegetable lo mein; vegetable kabobs; bean tacos, burritos or nachos; veggie or black-bean burgers; lentil-based soups and stews; and soy cheese and crackers.

- Choose vitamin-fortified breakfast cereals.

- Enjoy a variety of fresh, frozen, canned and dried fruits and vegetables every day.

- Add beans, peas, other legumes, nuts and seeds to salads to boost the protein content.

- Choose restaurants that offer a variety of vegetarian dishes. Vegetarian ethnic cuisine is easy to find; and you can choose from Chinese (egg foo yung or vegetable tofu stir fry), French (ratatouille or vegetable quiche), Indian (curried eggplant and potatoes), Italian (pasta primavera, eggplant Parmesan or involtini), Greek (spanakopita and tzatziki), Mexican (bean burrito and chiles rellenos) and Middle Eastern (falafel, hummus and tabouli), among others.

- Order salads, soups, breads and fruits if a restaurant doesn't offer vegetarian dishes.

- When traveling, call the airline at least 48 hours in advance to ask for a vegetarian meal.

grocery shopping tips*

Bring balanced nutrition into your home by following the MyPyramid Shopping Checklist below. In addition, remember to read food labels, and follow these tips:

- **Pay attention to serving size and servings per container.** If you consume one serving, the label clearly outlines the nutrients you'll obtain. If you double the serving, you double the calories and nutrients.

- **Read the ingredients list.** What are you eating? Look right below the Nutrition Facts Panel and find out. Skip items that include partially hydrogenated oils (trans fat), lots of added sugars or caloric sweeteners and sodium.

- **Make your calories count.** Look at the calories on the label as well as the nutrients the products provide. Is it a nutrient-dense or calorie-dense item? Compare items, and choose the one with the most nutrients for the fewest calories.

- **Know your fats.** Look for items low in saturated fats, trans fats and cholesterol. Remember 5% DV is low; 20% DV is high. Aim for most of your fats to come from unsaturated sources (mono- and polyunsaturated).

- **Say "Good-bye sodium"; say "Hello potassium."** Surprisingly, most sodium comes from processed foods, not from the saltshaker! Reduce your intake of prepackaged meals high in sodium (most microwave meals). Choose reduced-sodium options; and stock up on foods high in potassium (such as tomatoes, bananas, potatoes and orange juice), which counteract some of sodium's adverse effects on blood pressure.

* *Although this is a well-rounded grocery list, it is not exhaustive. Use it as a general guide, but feel free to include additional healthy choices that may not be listed here.*

Dairy

- ❑ skim, $1/2$% or 1% milk
- ❑ low-fat, part-skim or reduced-fat cheeses
- ❑ fat-free or reduced-fat yogurt
- ❑ fat-free or reduced-fat sour cream
- ❑ fat-free or reduced-fat cream cheese or Neufchatel cheese
- ❑ _____

Breads, Muffins and Rolls

- ❑ yeast breads (whole-wheat, rye, pumpernickel, multi-grain, raisin)
- ❑ whole-wheat bagels and pitas
- ❑ English muffins
- ❑ corn tortillas (baked)
- ❑ low-fat flour tortillas
- ❑ fat-free or low-fat biscuit mix
- ❑ _____

Cereals, Crackers, Rice and Pasta

- ❑ whole-grain cereals, dry or cooked (look for 3 g fiber or more and 10 g sugar or less per serving)
- ❑ graham crackers
- ❑ wasa crackers
- ❑ low-fat, low-sodium snack crackers
- ❑ rice (brown, wild and white)
- ❑ pasta (whole-wheat)
- ❑ bulgur, couscous and kasha
- ❑ potato mixes (made without fat)
- ❑ hominy
- ❑ polenta
- ❑ quinoa
- ❑ millet
- ❑ oatmeal
- ❑ aramanth
- ❑ polvillo
- ❑ tabouli grain salad
- ❑ _____

Meat

- ❑ white meat chicken and turkey (skinless)
- ❑ fish (not battered)
- ❑ scallops
- ❑ beef, round or sirloin
- ❑ extra-lean ground beef
- ❑ pork tenderloin
- ❑ 95% fat-free lunch meats or low-fat deli meats
- ❑ eggs or egg substitute
- ❑ tofu
- ❑ _____

Fruit (fresh, frozen and canned in water)

- ❑ apples
- ❑ applesauce (no sugar added)
- ❑ bananas
- ❑ blueberries
- ❑ raspberries
- ❑ strawberries
- ❑ peaches
- ❑ oranges
- ❑ pears
- ❑ grapes
- ❑ grapefruit
- ❑ apricots
- ❑ dried fruits
- ❑ cherries
- ❑ plums
- ❑ melons
- ❑ lemons
- ❑ limes
- ❑ plantains
- ❑ mangoes
- ❑ kiwi
- ❑ olives
- ❑ figs
- ❑ currants
- ❑ persimmons

- ❑ pineapple
- ❑ pomegranates
- ❑ quinces
- ❑ papaya
- ❑ zapote
- ❑ guava
- ❑ starfruit
- ❑ 100-percent fruit juice
  (no sugar added)
- ❑ _____

- ❑ mustard greens
- ❑ kale
- ❑ leeks
- ❑ bamboo shoots
- ❑ Chinese celery
- ❑ bok choy
- ❑ napa cabbage
- ❑ seaweed
- ❑ rhubarb
- ❑ _____

Vegetables (fresh, frozen and canned, low-sodium or no-salt-added)

- ❑ broccoli
- ❑ spinach
- ❑ salad mix
- ❑ summer/winter squash
- ❑ green beans
- ❑ romaine lettuce
- ❑ cabbage
- ❑ artichokes
- ❑ corn
- ❑ cauliflower
- ❑ cucumber
- ❑ asparagus
- ❑ mushrooms
- ❑ celery
- ❑ carrots
- ❑ onions
- ❑ sweet potatoes
- ❑ other potatoes
- ❑ fresh tomatoes
- ❑ stewed, diced tomatoes
- ❑ tomato sauce
- ❑ green, red or yellow bell peppers
- ❑ chilies
- ❑ vegetable medley (frozen)
- ❑ eggplant
- ❑ okra
- ❑ grape leaves

Beans and Legumes (if canned, no-salt-added)

- ❑ lentils
- ❑ black beans
- ❑ red/kidney beans
- ❑ navy beans
- ❑ pinto beans
- ❑ black-eyed peas
- ❑ fava beans
- ❑ Italian white beans
- ❑ great white northern beans
- ❑ chickpeas (garbanzo beans)
- ❑ peas
- ❑ _____

Nuts and Seeds (unsalted)

- ❑ almonds
- ❑ peanuts
- ❑ pecans
- ❑ cashews
- ❑ walnuts
- ❑ sesame seeds
- ❑ pumpkin seeds
- ❑ sunflower seeds
- ❑ flaxseeds (ground)
- ❑ nut butters (low saturated fat,
  low sugar)
- ❑ _____

Baking Items

- ❑ flour, all-purpose and whole-wheat
- ❑ sugar, brown, white or powdered
- ❑ nonstick cooking spray
- ❑ canned evaporated fat-free milk
- ❑ nonfat dry milk powder
- ❑ cocoa powder, unsweetened
- ❑ baking powder and soda
- ❑ cornstarch
- ❑ gelatin (sugar-free)
- ❑ pudding (sugar-free)
- ❑ angel food cake/mix
- ❑ _____

Frozen Foods

- ❑ microwave meals (low-sodium, low-fat)
- ❑ sorbet
- ❑ frozen yogurt
- ❑ whole-wheat dough
- ❑ _____

Condiments, Sauces and Seasonings

- ❑ fat-free or low-fat salad dressings
- ❑ mustard
- ❑ catsup
- ❑ barbecue sauce
- ❑ jams and jelly made with fruit, less sugar added
- ❑ spices
- ❑ herbs
- ❑ flavored vinegars (balsamic)
- ❑ plum sauce
- ❑ salsa or picante
- ❑ soy sauce (low-sodium)
- ❑ marinades (low-sodium)
- ❑ bouillon cubes/granules (low-sodium)
- ❑ chicken, beef and vegetable broth (low-fat, low-sodium)
- ❑ _____

Beverages

- ❑ no-calorie drink mixes
- ❑ unsweetened iced tea
- ❑ carbonated water
- ❑ bottled water
- ❑ 100-percent fruit and vegetable juices (no sugar added)
- ❑ _____

Fats and Oils

- ❑ olive oil
- ❑ canola oil
- ❑ safflower oil
- ❑ flaxseed oil
- ❑ peanut oil
- ❑ mayonnaise (low-fat)
- ❑ soft (tub, squeeze or spray), trans-fat-free margarine
- ❑ _____

the fitness top 10!

Most of us have read countless news reports about the value of exercise and the role it plays in our quest for better health. New studies continually point to the health benefits of exercise. You can move steadily toward increasing your health and ensure that physical activity becomes a consistent part of your lifestyle by following the practical tips of the Fitness Top 10.

1. Progress Wisely
Exercising too much and too vigorously is a common mistake that often results in injury. Rest after exercise, and gradually progress in time and intensity; this is the best way to develop a routine that you will look forward to and not abandon.

2. Add Variety
Too many people find a routine or physical activity they like and then never vary from it. Doing the same workout every day can lead to boredom—one of the top four reasons why people quit.

3. Set Realistic Goals
Unrealistic and vaguely stated goals lead to exercise dropout. It's important to establish a training goal that is specific and appropriate for your fitness and skill levels (do something a bit challenging but not overly difficult).

4. Make Physical Activity an Appointment
Those who fail to plan, plan to fail. Plan a daily time for your workout, but be flexible so that you can adjust when life interrupts your plan.

5. Do Something Every Day
Not having a full hour to exercise is no reason to skip your workout. Research shows that even three 10-minute exercise sessions a day can provide important health benefits.

6. Find a Buddy

Studies show that those who exercise with a friend or group find more success and accountability. Your participation will also motivate a friend to get moving.

7. Invest in the Proper Shoes and Equipment

Using outdated, improper or old gear, such as the walking shoes you've worn for three years, puts you at risk for injury. An investment in good shoes and other equipment will motivate you and keep you injury free.

8. Learn from Past Failures and Successes

So many of us are unwilling to try for fear of failure. If you previously dropped out of an exercise program, it probably wasn't the right one for you. Try again, and evaluate your new routine as you progress.

9. Expect to Become Weary

It's normal to come out of the gate running for about the first two weeks, and then *bam!* The new wears off, the honeymoon is over, and your workout is nothing but hard work. What do you do then? The answer is simple. When you start your new program, *expect the newness to wear off.* We all become weary; but if you stay diligent and press on, you will reap wonderful benefits!

10. Celebrate Appropriately   8/8/10

Reward yourself as you reach goals along the way: Do something special after you've walked your first mile, run your first race, attended your first water-aerobics class. Good rewards might be a pair of new workout shoes, new workout clothes or a trip to your favorite getaway.

I need to reward myself for being faithful to my workout – almost daily.

1. Swimsuit
2. Shoes
3. resistance board

I have to find something in Sept.

the benefits of
physical activity!

When was the last time you took a walk or engaged in some sort of activity that got your blood pumping? Perhaps you exercised for a time but got out of the routine. Did you know that 75 percent of people who start an exercise program drop out within the first three to six months? Yet *physical activity is as important to overall health as nutrition.* The truth is, if you make physical activity part of your lifestyle, you will not only feel better, but you will also be more successful at losing pounds or maintaining your goal weight.

If you've become a couch potato in recent years or months, you're invited right now to begin wherever you are and get moving once again. If you're not sure where to start or if you just need some motivation, read on! The information in this section will help you take some first steps toward healthy, positive change.

The following abbreviated list of benefits serves as a good starting point. If you have a family history of a chronic disease, pay close attention to the merits of consistent exercise. If you experience mood swings, notice how exercise can positively impact your emotions. The list below includes something for everyone! Determine which benefits most interest you, and why; then plan how to include daily physical activity in your life.

- **Exercise is good for your heart.** Even 30 minutes of moderate-intensity activity (think about walking as if you're late for an appointment, for example) most days of the week can help prevent heart disease. The heart muscle is essential for pumping oxygen-rich blood to your major muscle groups and organs. Not only does regular activity strengthen your heart muscle, but it also lowers blood pressure, increases the good (or HDL) cholesterol, lowers the bad (or LDL) cholesterol, and enhances blood flow. These benefits reduce your risk of stroke, heart disease and high blood pressure. Amazingly, studies have shown that you can get the same benefit from three 10-minute bouts of moderate activity each day as you do from one 30-minute session.

- **Exercise plays a role in preventing cancer.** At least 35 percent of all cancer deaths may be related to weight issues and lack of activity. Studies have shown that regular activity helps lower the risk of cancers of the colon, prostate, uterine lining and breast.

- **Exercise reduces the risk for developing type-2 diabetes.** More than 17 million Americans have type-2 diabetes (the number of people diagnosed is increasing epidemically and now includes children), which affects the way your body uses blood sugar. A study published in the *Annals of Internal Medicine* found that a brisk walk for one hour each day can reduce the risk of type-2 diabetes by 34 percent.

- **Exercise promotes weight loss.** It's no secret that exercise burns calories. Fitness expert Bob Greene, known for his work with Oprah Winfrey, refers to activity as "the gift that keeps on giving." Why? It raises your metabolism for a few hours after you've stopped exercising; thus, the rate at which you burn calories will remain higher than normal. Research has shown that to have the greatest effect on weight loss, you need to reduce your caloric intake and increase your exercise. The type of exercise or activity is not nearly as important as being persistent until consistent.

- **Exercise helps improve muscle strength, joint structure and joint function.** A certain level of muscle strength is needed for everyday activities such as walking and climbing stairs. Through strength training, you can increase not only your muscle strength and muscle mass but also your bone strength.

- **Exercise prevents osteoporosis.** Strength training and weight-bearing activities, together with a healthy calcium intake, build strong bones. Exercise with impact (such as running, walking and lifting weights) helps combat and even reverse the signs of osteoporosis. The Nurses' Health Study revealed that women who walked four or more hours a week had 41 percent fewer hip fractures than those who walked less than an hour a week.

- **Exercise provides emotional benefits.** Need a psychological lift? Physical activity impacts your body's norepinephrine and serotonin levels. These are neurotransmitters that are involved in how you react to daily events. Exercise also causes your body to release feel-good chemicals called endorphins. If you want to de-stress or improve your mood, consider taking your dog for a brisk walk. It may change the course of your day.

- **Exercise battles the effects of aging.** Recent literature suggests that the greatest threat to health is not the aging process itself but, rather, inactivity. Exercise helps provide a better quality of life in many ways. In addition to warding off numerous chronic diseases, regular exercise slows down the degeneration of the central nervous system, which leads to slower reaction times and poor coordination. In a Harvard study, men who burned at least 2,000 calories a week by walking, jogging, climbing stairs or playing sports lived one to two years longer on average than did those who burned fewer than 500 calories a week by exercising.

- **Exercise promotes brain health.** Scientists believe that exercise increases the flow of blood to the brain, just as it improves circulation to the heart and the rest of the body. Activity also stimulates the growth of nerve cells in the part of the brain involved in memory. Researchers from the University of Illinois found that the brain responses in active seniors were comparable to those of young adults.

- **Exercise prevents colds.** Researchers from the University of North Carolina found that people who exercised regularly were 23 percent less likely to get colds than those who exercised less. Moreover, when those who exercised got colds, the symptoms disappeared more quickly than in the study participants who did little exercise. Health experts believe that exercise spikes the immune system for a few hours each day, helping ward off colds.

- **Exercise improves sleeping patterns.** Physical activity releases God's natural tranquilizers, called endorphins. If you're having problems going to sleep or if your sleep is typically interrupted, try to exercise at least three hours before bedtime in order to improve your chances of a restful sleep.

- **Exercise enhances your sex life.** How could we leave it out? Experts confirm that the fitter we are, the better our sex life is. According to the American Council on Exercise, being physically active can be "a natural Viagra boost." Being fit improves libido, blood circulation and sexual function. It also may make you feel better about yourself and, as a result, more sexually inclined.

After reviewing these benefits, indicate below which ones motivate you to get active.

_____

_____

_____

_____

_____

_____

_____

_____

Deciding that you're going to lead a more active lifestyle is just the beginning of a new life of health and energy! The information in "Starting a Basic Exercise Program" (the next article in this guide) will help you take your first steps toward this life of health and energy and make the changes you need to discover a new quality of life.

starting a basic
exercise program!

How many times have you started an exercise program only to quit after a few weeks of frustration and soreness? Most people give up on exercise routines because of time restraints, lack of results, injury or boredom. Which of these have slowed you down in the past? First Place 4 Health wants to help you find just the right activity mode that will work for you and fit your lifestyle. Our goal is to encourage you to focus on the way exercise makes you feel at the end of a session and to enjoy the results and benefits of exercise on your health and well-being. We will provide tools for you to be successful on your fitness journey regardless of your fitness level. Throughout the next few chapters, you will see two shaded sidebars:

BEGINNING WITH A LOT TO LOSE
and
GOING THE EXTRA MILE

In the following pages, you'll find hints just for you and where you are on your fitness journey.

BEGINNING WITH A LOT TO LOSE

Beginning with a Lot to Lose are suggestions for those of you who are deconditioned, are just beginning to exercise, are recovering from an injury, or have a lot of weight to lose. Use wisdom and discuss your exercise plan with your doctor, whether or not you have any medical concerns.

GOING THE EXTRA MILE

Going the Extra Mile are tips for those of you who have been regularly exercising and would like to achieve a higher level of fitness.

PROGRAMMED ACTIVITY VERSUS LIFESTYLE ACTIVITY

The First Place 4 Health fitness philosophy for exercise is simple: *Something is better than nothing, and more is better than less.* Recent studies show that even a small amount of activity can have lasting health benefits.

For most of us, becoming more physically active means taking intentional steps to incorporate activity into our daily lifestyles.

You may notice that experts rarely use the word "exercise." Instead, they focus on "activity." That's right! You don't have to exercise to get many of the health benefits associated with physical activity.

Physical activity does not have to be programmed into your already busy schedule. Programmed exercise—attending a fitness class, brisk walking, jogging, aerobic dance, bicycling or swimming—offers numerous health benefits. But there are many other physical activities that performed daily also provide long-term health and fitness benefits. Examples include mowing the lawn, taking the stairs instead of the elevator, parking in the last space so that you'll have to walk farther, and planting a garden. *Small lifestyle changes that increase moderate-intensity physical activity are as effective as a structured exercise program in improving long-term cardiovascular fitness and blood pressure.*

The best activity to help you meet your fitness goals is *one that you will do*. First Place 4 Health recommends that you combine lifestyle activity with a programmed activity for even greater variety and benefits.

COMPONENTS OF A BALANCED PROGRAM

A balanced exercise program should include the following components:

- Cardiovascular exercises
- Strength-training exercises
- Flexibility and balance exercises
- A record of your BMI (body mass index)

BETTER LATE THAN NEVER

A study published in *The Journal of the American Medical Association* reveals that it is never too late to reap the health benefits of physical activity. Inactive women age 65 and older who began walking a mile a day cut their rate of death from all causes by 50 percent.

The words "cardiovascular system" refer to your heart and blood vessels. *Cardiovascular exercises* strengthen your lungs and heart and enhance weight loss by helping you burn calories. *Strength-training exercises* promote muscular strength and endurance, help prevent injury, and increase lean-muscle mass. Strength training can improve your strength and posture, reduce the risk of lower-back injury and help you stay toned. The more muscle you have, the more calories you burn each day. *Flexibility exercises* are needed to maintain joint range of motion and reduce the risk of injury and muscle soreness. *Balance exercises* strengthen your core body muscles and help you develop your sense of balance, which diminishes as we age.

Your *BMI,* a measure of body fat based on height and weight that applies to both adult men and women, should be recorded periodically so that your progress can be tracked. Your goal is to get your BMI into the normal range. (How to measure your BMI was addressed earlier in the "Your Health Assessment" article.)

GUIDELINES TO KEEP IN MIND

- Set a long-term goal of incorporating four physical activity recommendations (discussed in the following articles) into your lifestyle.

- Choose the recommendations and level of activity that are right for you, and remember that you do not need to start all components at once.

- Increase the frequency, duration and number of days, adding in the other recommendations (for example, strength training) as you become ready.

- Set realistic short-term goals and start slowly.

In general, during *moderate activity*, you should feel like you are pushing yourself somewhat or working with a purpose. Your pace should cause some increase in breathing but not so much that you can't carry on a conversation. You should feel back to normal within 30 minutes of working out.

If you can't spend 30 uninterrupted minutes working out, remember that three 10-minute periods of activity during the day are just as beneficial. You will not have time for a 5- to 10-minute warm-up and cool-down, so begin your activity at a slower pace, then speed up in the middle and slow down toward the end.

When you begin an extended period of activity (30 minutes or more), always begin with a *warm-up*. A warm-up consists of 5 to 10 minutes of light activity and stretching. A warm-up will gradually increase your heart rate and breathing and loosen your muscles and joints for activity. This will make your activity more enjoyable and lower your risk of injury.

End moderate to vigorous activity with a *cool-down*. A cool-down consists of 5 to 10 minutes of light activity and stretching. It will gradually slow down your heart rate and breathing and help keep your muscles and joints loose following activity. This may be the best time to do flexibility activities because the muscles and joints are warm and loose.

the FITT formula for exercise

First Place 4 Health encourages lifestyle activity for its many health benefits. However, for those of you who are interested in programmed activity, the FITT formula for exercise—Frequency, Intensity, Time, Type—will be your guide.

Frequency answers the question "How often should I exercise?"
Intensity answers the question "How hard should I exercise?"
Time answers the question "How long should I exercise?"
Type answers the question "What kind of exercises should I do?"

The FITT formula works in the components of a balanced fitness program: cardiovascular exercises, strength-training exercises, and flexibility and balance exercises.

CARDIOVASCULAR EXERCISES

Frequency: 3 to 5 days a week
Intensity: 50 percent to 85 percent of target heart rate
Time: 20 to 60 minutes of continuous aerobic activity (minimum of 10-minute bouts accumulated throughout the day)
Type: Activities that use large muscle groups, can be maintained continuously and are aerobic in nature

STRENGTH-TRAINING EXERCISES

Frequency: 2 to 3 days per week
Intensity: A minimum of one set of 8 to 12 repetitions on each muscle group to the point of muscle fatigue
Time: 20 to 30 minutes for most individuals

Type: Separate exercises that use resistance to strengthen major muscle groups—arms, shoulders, core body, and legs; usually includes the use of free weights, circuit training, resistance bands and/or body weight

FLEXIBILITY AND BALANCE EXERCISES

Frequency: Daily
Intensity: Gentle stretching to the point of tension, never pain
Time: 10 minutes, holding each stretch 10 to 30 seconds
Type: General stretches of all major muscle groups and tendons

As you become more active and fit, try for a daily combination of both lifestyle activity and programmed activity.

TURN OFF THE TUBE

A simple way to get off the couch and lose a few pounds at the same time is to turn off your TV. A recent study of the habits involving 5,000 National Weight Control Registry members (people who have lost an average of 73 pounds and have kept off at least 30 pounds for more than 6 years) revealed that most of them watch fewer than 10 hours of television a week. The national average of TV viewing per week is a whopping 28 hours.

the activity pyramid

Experts tell us there are many ways to get the benefits of a physically active lifestyle. A variety of daily activities provide the foundation for good health. The activity pyramid, based on the recommendations of major health and fitness organizations, illustrates a balanced and healthy plan for daily physical activity. It's a simple guide for visualizing how physical activity can fit into your life. You can use this guide to choose what works best for you based on your goals, interests and abilities.

LEVELS OF THE PYRAMID

Lifestyle Activities

The base of the pyramid includes lifestyle activities that can easily fit into your daily routine. The good news is that lifestyle activities don't have to be done all at one time. Short periods of activity will result in health benefits as long as the total of the periods adds up to 30 minutes or more each day. Lifestyle activities such as walking, climbing the stairs, doing housework, playing with the kids and leisure bicycling are great ways to get started on a program of healthy physical activity.

What lifestyle activities are you ready to add to your day?

_____

_____

_____

_____

_____

THE ACTIVITY PYRAMID

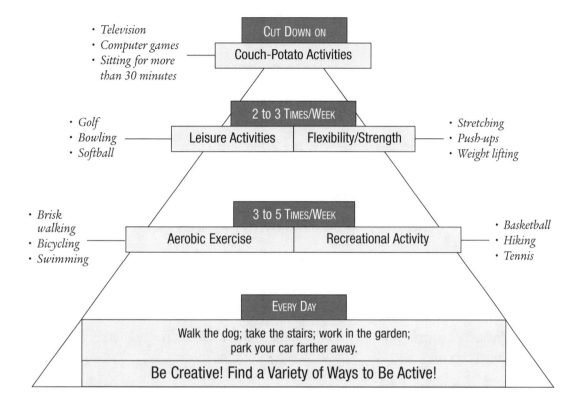

Aerobic Activities

The next level of the pyramid includes aerobic activities. This level follows the more traditional FITT prescription. Because aerobic activities are typically more vigorous, 20 minutes at least 3 days each week will provide benefits similar to those of daily lifestyle activities. As the variety, intensity and duration of activities increase, the health and fitness benefits increase. The more active you are, the more calories you burn.

Strength and Flexibility Activities

The third level of the pyramid emphasizes strength and flexibility exercises. Muscular strength and endurance are also important for overall health and quality of life. Strong muscles allow you to participate in a variety of daily activities with ease and enjoyment. Strength-building activities should be performed two to three days each week. Performing one set of several different exercises that use all the major muscle groups is all you need. You can use your own body weight, elastic bands or small hand-weights. Flexibility is the ability to move the joints through a full range of motion. It reduces pain and stiffness, prevents injuries and makes you feel better. Flexibility exercises should be performed every day, but a minimum of two to three days each week is acceptable.

DESIGN YOUR OWN PROGRAM

Now that you know the components of a balanced exercise program, you are ready to begin designing your own.

- Choose activities in each of these categories that are based on your own personal goals and interests.

- Start with enjoyable activities that fit easily into your lifestyle.

- Start slowly and make regular activity a habit. Strive to be active every day.

- If you're having trouble getting started, look for ways to cut down on the time you spend in sedentary activities.

- Challenge yourself to get up and move, even if it's just for a few minutes.

- Once physical activity becomes an enjoyable habit, look for new opportunities to fit activity into your day.

- Add flexibility and strength exercises when you're ready.

- Consider activities such as hiking, skiing, golf, a local fun run and other recreational activities.

- Set a long-term goal of doing physical activities from each level of the pyramid every week. This is an enjoyable way to achieve total body conditioning.

SET AN EXAMPLE

About 65 percent of adults in the United States are considered overweight or obese, and 31 percent are overweight or at risk of becoming so. Physically active parents can serve as positive role models and influence their children's overall quality of life.

cardiovascular
exercises

ardiovascular exercises are designed to strengthen your heart and lungs and help you burn excess calories. By now, you have decided on a calorie range for your food intake. Combining that reduction in calories with the calories you will be burning with daily cardio exercises will help you reduce body fat.

You will also experience many additional health benefits as the variety, intensity and duration of activities increase. To improve your cardiovascular endurance, try activities that keep your heart rate elevated at a safe level for a sustained length of time, such as walking, swimming or bicycling. The activity you choose does not have to be strenuous to improve your cardiovascular endurance. Start slowly with an activity you enjoy, and gradually work up to a more intense pace. For every hour of moderate physical activity that modern conveniences replace, you lose 200 to 300 calories. Actually, experts estimate that Americans use 500 fewer calories per day then they did 100 years ago.

Cardiovascular activity and increased lifestyle activity both burn calories. The following chart shows the estimated number of calories that a 150-pound person burns while performing a variety of exercises for one hour. The numbers vary depending on your weight, your body composition and the level of intensity of the activity. (As a frame of reference, sleep burns 45 calories an hour.)

ACTIVITY	CALORIES BURNED PER HOUR	ACTIVITY	CALORIES BURNED PER HOUR
Biking	441	Strolling	206
Cleaning, Heavy	432	Swimming	603
Cleaning, Light	240	Tennis	549
Dancing	370	Vacuuming/Mopping	150
Gardening	324	Walking, Brisk	297
Jogging	675	Yoga	360
Mowing Lawn	324		

(Source: American Cancer Society. Calories burned per hour are based on a 150-pound individual.)

As you prepare to improve your cardiovascular endurance, ask yourself these questions:

1 *What activities would I enjoy?*

2 *Am I ready to add these activities into my week?*

3 *When will I do it?*

4 *Who can help me get started?*

WALKING PROGRAMS

First Place 4 Health recommends walking as one of the easiest ways to get fit.

For most of us, walking comes as naturally as breathing—that is, until we wake up and discover that we can't do it like we used to. For some people with health and weight issues, even walking the shortest distance is a challenge. Regardless of your fitness level, walking is still a great place to start. It is inexpensive, can be done anywhere and doesn't require practice or special equipment. According to a recent study by the U.S. Centers for Disease Control and Prevention, the most popular exercise for individuals wanting to lose weight is walking. Here's how various activities stack up for men and women:

Men	Women
Walking—37.7 percent	Walking—52.5 percent
Running and jogging—10.7 percent	Aerobics—8.7 percent
Weight lifting—9.6 percent	Gardening—8.2 percent
Golfing—8.1 percent	Exercise machines—8 percent

First Place 4 Health recommends two tried-and-true walking programs: 10,000 Steps a Day and the 100-Mile Club. These programs will help keep you motivated and provide a tool for self-evaluation and accountability.

10,000 Steps a Day

Working toward 10,000 steps a day is a wonderful way to increase lifestyle activity without having to program or calendar in the exercise time. Recent studies show the following benefits of 10,000 steps a day:

- **Walking helps prevent heart disease in women.** According to the American Heart Association, heart disease is on the decline in men but on the increase in women.

Women are six times more likely to die from heart disease than breast cancer, and heart disease kills more women over age 65 than any other disease.

- **Walking provides an incentive to increase activity levels.** In a recent study, participants who monitored their daily steps with pedometers tended to walk more every day, even when they were below their goal of 10,000 steps per day.

- **Walking helps improve overall body composition.** Middle-aged women who took at least 10,000 steps per day on average were much more likely to fall into recommended ranges for total body weight and body fat percentage, according to the results of a study published in *Medicine and Science in Sports and Exercise.* Conversely, inactive women—those taking fewer than 6,000 steps per day—were more likely to be overweight or obese and have a higher waist circumference, which increases the risk of cardiovascular disease.

Determine Your Walking Category. Most sedentary Americans move only about 2,000 to 3,000 steps a day. Studies reveal that increasing the number up to 6,000 steps a day can significantly reduce the risk of death, and 8,000 to 10,000 steps a day promotes weight loss. Wear a pedometer for a week, and determine which of the following categories describes you:

- 5,000 or fewer steps a day: sedentary
- 5,000 to 7,499 steps a day: low active
- 7,500 to 9,999 steps a day: somewhat active (likely to include some exercise or walking)
- 10,000 steps a day: active or moderately active
- 12,500 or more steps a day: highly active

STEP EQUIVALENTS	
1 mile	2,100 average steps
1 block	200 average steps
10 minutes of walking	1,200 steps on average
bicycling or swimming	150 steps per minute
weight lifting	100 steps per minute
roller-skating	200 steps per minute

(Source: www.about.com.)

Make Every Step Count with a Pedometer. A pedometer is a simple device you wear (generally above your hip) that counts the number of steps you take. It tracks your steps by detecting body motion, so even small steps can speed you toward your fitness goals. Pedometers are relatively inexpensive but may have more features than you actually need. To get the most mileage out of a pedometer, keep these hints in mind:

- Choose a pedometer with a large display screen that is easy to read and has a clip that stays snugly against your body and won't easily slip or bounce off. A safety strap is a nice feature.

- Establish a baseline of steps by measuring the number of steps you take in an average day. To determine your baseline standard, record your findings for three days, add them up and divide by three.

- Increase your steps gradually (approximately 200 to 1,000 steps a day) by adding to your baseline average.

- Your goal will be 10,000 steps a day, which is approximately 5 miles. The pedometer may record all body movement, so turn it off when you are not taking steps.

To ensure that you wear your pedometer, keep it in a prominent place, such as your bathroom counter, so that you will remember to snap it on every morning.

The 100-Mile Club

Can't walk that mile yet? Don't be discouraged! There are exercises you can do to strengthen your body and burn those extra calories. Just keep moving!

You will be surprised at how quickly your activity adds up each month. The key is to be consistent. Keep a record of your activity minutes on your Live It Tracker or in your Bible study (the 100-mile chart on the inside back cover). Then convert those minutes to miles, following the chart below. You are not competing with anyone but yourself. Your job is to strive to reach 100 miles before the last meeting in your current First Place 4 Health group session.

Walking

slowly, 2 mph	30 min. = 156 cal. = 1 mile
moderately, 3 mph	20 min. = 156 cal. = 1 mile
very briskly, 4 mph	15 min. = 156 cal. = 1 mile
speed walking	10 min. = 156 cal. = 1 mile
up stairs	13 min. = 159 cal. = 1 mile

Running/Jogging
10 min. = 156 cal. = 1 mile

Cycling Outdoors

slowly, < 10 mph	20 min. = 156 cal. = 1 mile

light effort, 10-12 mph   12 min. = 156 cal. = 1 mile
moderate effort, 12-14 mph.   10 min. = 156 cal. = 1 mile
vigorous effort, 14-16 mph   7.5 min. = 156 cal. = 1 mile
very fast, 16-19 mph   6.5 min. = 152 cal. = 1 mile

Sports Activities

Playing tennis (singles)   10 min. = 156 cal. = 1 mile
Swimming
   light to moderate effort   11 min. = 152 cal. = 1 mile
   fast, vigorous effort   7.5 min. = 156 cal. = 1 mile
Softball   15 min. = 156 cal. = 1 mile
Golf   20 min. = 156 cal. = 1 mile
Rollerblading   6.5 min. = 152 cal. = 1 mile
Ice skating   11 min. = 152 cal. = 1 mile
Jumping rope   7.5 min. = 156 cal. = 1 mile
Basketball   12 min. = 156 cal. = 1 mile
Soccer (casual)   15 min. = 159 cal. = 1 mile

Around the House

Mowing grass   22 min. = 156 cal. = 1 mile
Mopping, sweeping, vacuuming   19.5 min. = 155 cal. = 1 mile
Cooking   40 min. =160 cal. = 1 mile
Gardening   19 min. = 156 cal. = 1 mile
Housework (general)   35 min. = 156 cal. = 1 mile
Ironing   45 min. = 153 cal. = 1 mile
Raking leaves   25 min. = 150 cal. = 1 mile
Washing car   23 min. = 156 cal. = 1 mile
Washing dishes   45 min. = 153 cal. = 1 mile

At the Gym

Stair machine   8.5 min. = 155 cal. = 1 mile
Stationary bike
   slowly, 10 mph   30 min. = 156 cal. = 1 mile
   moderately, 10-13 mph   15 min. = 156 cal. = 1 mile
   vigorously, 13-16 mph   7.5 min. = 156 cal. = 1 mile
   briskly, 16-19 mph   6.5 min. = 156 cal. = 1 mile
Elliptical trainer   12 min. = 156 cal. = 1 mile
Weight machines (used vigorously)   13 min. = 152 cal.=1 mile
Aerobics
   low impact   15 min. = 156 cal. = 1 mile
   high impact   12 min. = 156 cal. = 1 mile
   water   20 min. = 156 cal. = 1 mile
Pilates   15 min. = 156 cal. = 1 mile
Raquetball (casual)   15 min. = 159 cal. = 1 mile
Stretching exercises   25 min. = 150 cal. = 1 mile
Weight lifting (would also work   30 min. = 156 cal. = 1 mile
   for weight machines used
   moderately or gently)

Family Leisure

Playing piano	37 min. = 155 cal. = 1 mile
Jumping rope	10 min. = 152 cal. = 1 mile
Skating (moderate)	20 min. = 152 cal. = 1 mile
Swimming	
moderate	17 min. = 156 cal. = 1 mile
vigorous	10 min. = 148 cal. = 1 mile
Table tennis	25 min. = 150 cal. = 1 mile
Walk/run/play with kids	25 min. = 150 cal. = 1 mile

GET STARTED WITH A WALKING PROGRAM

To get started with either of the walking programs—10,000 Steps a Day or the 100-Mile Club—is easy, and there are only a few basic things that you'll need:

1 **A good pair of walking shoes.** Walking shoes do not have to be expensive, but they do need to have a lot of stability and plenty of space in the toe box for wiggle room.

2 **Appropriate undergarments.** If your thighs rub together, you might want to consider a pair of lycra bike shorts or leggings to help prevent chafing. A good sports bra is also a necessity for large-busted women.

3 **Pedometer.** A pedometer is optional, but you'll find that tracking your progress is so much easier if you have one.

4 **Positive attitude.** A positive attitude in not an option—it is mandatory!

Using a pedometer or logging your miles will help keep you accountable. Those numbers don't lie! To maximize your walking program, consider the following suggestions:

- When you take walks, go to the end of the sidewalk and all the away around the cul-de-sac—no shortcuts!

- Walk while you talk on the phone. Keep a steady pace.

- Use your small chunks of time. If you only have 10 minutes, use them wisely! Three 10-minute walks have the same health benefits as one 30-minute walk.

- Keep an extra pair of walking shoes in the car. Take advantage of situations when you are stuck somewhere.

- Get out of the car. Don't wait in the car when you are picking up your child from practice. Arrive early and walk.

■ Make your walk an extension of your quiet time. After completing your Bible study, head out the door for your prayer time.

HOW TO BUY ATHLETIC SHOES

■ Shop late in the day when your feet are their largest (feet swell during the day).

■ Measure your foot while standing, and make sure you have enough room in the toe box to curl your toes up without discomfort.

■ Choose shoes that are comfortable immediately. If they hurt in the store, don't buy them.

■ Buy shoes that are designed for the exercise you are doing. Running shoes are not necessarily the best for aerobics or cross training. Running shoes can be fine for walking; but when you decide to start running, walking shoes may be too heavy.

■ If you are working out three times a week, you need to replace your shoes approximately every 500 miles or every six months.

■ If you have special needs, it may be worth your while to visit a store that specializes in custom fitting the athletic shoes you need to prevent injury. Wear your athletic shoes only for working out. They will last much longer if you don't wear them for everyday activities.

■ Buy two pairs of shoes if you find a style that really works for you. Styles are discontinued quickly.

■ Buy your next pair of shoes before your old pair wears out. Exercising in worn-out shoes can contribute to injuries. A new pair of shoes is a lot cheaper than knee surgery.

BEGINNING WITH A LOT TO LOSE

◆ **Start smart.** Begin with just 10 minutes a day, twice a day. Increase time slowly.

◆ **Start strong.** Support your feet to avoid injury. Foot pain is a common problem for beginners with a lot of weight to lose. Extra cushioning insoles in your walking shoes will help with impact and weight distribution.

GOING THE EXTRA MILE

- **Compete with yourself.** Increase your time one day and your distance the next.

- **Add a three-minute jog for every 15 minutes of walking.**

- **Enter and train for a walking half-marathon.** A half-marathon is almost the perfect race to train for. It's not nearly as time consuming as a full marathon but still presents a great challenge for the experienced walker. It consists of 13.1 miles and usually requires about 13 weeks of training. Seek a training group in your community.

- **Consider "Are You Ready to Run?"** if you're really up for a challenge (see *Simple Ideas for Healthy Living*). Running is an effective way to burn a lot of calories through exercise.

strength training

S trength training is a key element to any exercise program. It is important to note, however, that you should work at your own level and build gradually. Also, talk to your doctor before you begin your program, especially if you have high blood pressure or other health problems. Strength training doesn't replace cardiovascular exercise but enhances it because it works the muscles in a very different way. In fact, it is a great place to get started, because the stronger your muscles become, the easier it will be to participate in cardiovascular exercises.

There are numerous benefits of strength training:

1. *Strength training helps combat osteoporosis.* When you "stress" your skeletal muscles, you "stress" your skeleton. Bones become stronger and denser through strength training, as do the surrounding muscles.

2. *Strength training helps combat age-related problems and degenerative diseases.* Much of the bone and muscle loss that we attribute to aging is actually caused by lack of use.

3. *Strength training helps you tone.* Muscle weighs more than fat, but it takes up less space. As you develop strength, take your body measurements and be encouraged! Remember that muscle is the primary calorie burner. The more lean body tissue you have, the more calories you burn all day long!

4. *Strength training helps rehabilitate and strengthen previously injured or weak muscle groups.*

5. *Strength training can help correct muscle imbalances.* Two-thirds of all our muscles are located above our waist and are hardly touched by many popular aerobic activities.

6. *Strength training provides extra abdominal work.* When the abs are properly used to stabilize the torso during many weight-bearing exercises, your abdominal muscles get an extra workout.

7. ***Strength training makes many activities in everyday life easier.*** Improving your muscles and endurance will be reflected in your practical fitness as you go about your activities of daily living: lifting heavy grocery bags, picking up babies, moving furniture, and so forth.

HOW TO DEVELOP MUSCLE POWER

The American College of Sports Medicine recommends a minimum of two sessions of strength training per week. This is in addition to their recommendation of three to four sessions of cardio exercise (programmed activity) per week.

How much you get out of your strength-training workout is determined by three factors:

1 The number of times each movement is repeated (number of reps)

2 The speed of each movement

3 The size of the weights or the amount of resistance used

To train for strength rather than endurance, use *slower movements* and *heavier weights* or *stronger resistance bands*. (*Note:* Because women have different hormone levels than men, it is unlikely that women will see a dramatic increase in muscle size.) Select weights that are heavy enough to be a challenge. Strict strength training actually takes the muscle "to failure." This means that you cannot do another rep using proper form. Weights should be heavy enough that it is difficult to get through the entire set. As training begins, it may be necessary to stop and rest rather than continue. This is especially true if you start to compromise your position and compensate with other muscles groups such as the neck and back.

WHAT YOU NEED TO GET STARTED

First Place 4 Health recommends using handheld weights or resistance bands.

Handheld Weights

When using weights, work up to five-pound weights or more as quickly as possible to really experience the benefits of strength training. Even if you cannot do all the repetitions at first, you will see quick improvement by challenging your muscles with the heavier weights. Keep in mind that strength is lost quickly if you stop doing strength training (in other words, your muscles will atrophy). After a sickness, holiday or time away from strength training, you will have to build back up to the strength level you were at before.

Resistance Bands

Resistance bands are made of elastic, and most fitness stores have them available in several resistance sizes. They provide dynamic resistance through the whole range of motion of each exercise and can be very effective for strength cross-training because they challenge the muscle groups in a different way than hand weights. When using bands, always make sure you control the band and move through each exercise movement slowly in a controlled manner as the band provides external resistance.

KEYS TO PROPER STRENGTH TRAINING

1. *Keep a tight core body (tighten the abdominal and gluteus muscles) with every rep.* The key to proper alignment and execution of most strength-training movements is torso stabilization and good posture.

2. *Stop when you have performed all the reps you can do using proper form.* Proper body alignment is critical. Bad posture indicates fatigue. Do not compromise your position.

3. *Avoid hyperextension and locking joints.* Be especially mindful of your elbows and knees. If you lock a joint, then that joint (and not the muscles) is holding the weight. This doesn't build strength but leaves you open to injury by stressing the joint.

4. *Keep all movements slow and controlled.* Do not rush through any of the movements. Avoid heaving the weight and having to brake it at the end of the range of motion.

5. *Remember to breathe.* Exhale on exertion (when you are moving against gravity), and inhale on the release. Keep in mind that holding your breath can raise blood pressure.

6. *Work out at least two times per week.* The length of time for each session will vary and will depend on the number of muscle groups worked. Usually, a 30-minute session will be adequate time to target each muscle group. Once a week is not enough to see change. Three times a week may be even more effective; however, allow one day of rest between sessions so that your muscles can recover.

BEGINNING WITH A LOT TO LOSE

◆ Using free weights requires balance and control. Use only the size weight that you can control, beginning with five pounds or less. If you need help keeping your balance, hold on to the back of a chair with one hand.

◆ Protect areas of previous injury. Be particularly careful if you have had shoulder, neck or back injuries.

◆ If while working out you "feel" the exercises in the trapezius area of the neck and upper back, you may be using those muscles to compensate for weaker areas. If you feel pain in your neck or shoulders, try using lighter weights or doing fewer reps until you build strength.

◆ When lifting heavy weights above the head, it is extremely important to concentrate on abdominal stabilization.

◆ People with a lot to lose may have a limited range of motion because of excess body fat and girth, but this will not have a negative effect on the muscle group you are training.

◆ Shaking muscles are a sign that you are recruiting new muscle fibers. You are gaining strength, which is exactly what you want! As you become stronger, the shaking will decrease. Work through the shaking unless you are shaking to the point of compromising your stability.

GOING THE EXTRA MILE

◆ Consider adding a third day of strength training with a day of rest in between for recovery.

◆ Look into adding a Pilates core-body-strengthening class, or purchase a reputable Pilates DVD for home use.

flexibility and balance training!

Flexibility and balance are an important part of overall fitness, and both will improve with regular training. Flexibility, or stretching, exercises are one of the quickest ways to increase your fitness level. Benefits of flexibility training include (1) promotion and maintenance of range of motion in joints, (2) improvement of posture, (3) enhancement of physical and mental relaxation, (4) release of muscle tension and soreness, and (5) reduction of risk of injury.

Your level of flexibility is primarily tied to your genetics, gender, age and level of physical activity. Some people are naturally more flexible, but everyone can improve their flexibility with consistent exercise. Studies show that most loss of flexibility and balance is a result of inactivity rather than the aging process. The less active we are, the less flexible we are likely to be. Stretching and relaxation exercises can be modified for every fitness level.

FLEXIBILITY BASICS

Flexibility exercises, or stretches, are simple; but don't mistake simplicity for sloppiness. Every stretch should consist of three steps:

1 Start each stretch slowly, exhaling as you gently stretch the muscle.

2 Try to hold each stretch for at least 10 to 30 seconds.

3 Stretch all major muscles groups, paying closing attention to those that feel tight.

When stretching, avoid the following:

- Bouncing with the stretch (Bouncing causes short pulls on the muscle, actually keeping it from relaxing. The stretch will be more effective if you relax and ease into it.)

- Stretching a muscle that is not warmed up

- Holding your breath as you stretch

- Straining a muscle (Stretch to the point of tension, never pain.)

So many times before working out, it is tempting to skip the stretches to save time. The fact is, stretching warms up your muscles, lengthens them and gets them ready for action. You will run faster, throw better, jump higher, sit taller and feel better with a good stretch.

Just as you should stretch before you start your exercise program, you should take five minutes to stretch at the end of an exercise session. All cardiovascular exercise should be followed by at least a few minutes of stretching.

It's best to take a few minutes every day to stretch major muscle groups.

BALANCE AND STABILITY EXERCISES (BASE TRAINING)

Stability and balance training strengthens the core body muscles and improves balance. It also can aid in correcting poor posture. The muscles in your lower back, pelvis, hips and abdomen are all part of your core body. These muscles provide the support system for almost any activity or motion your body engages in, from sitting for long periods of time to walking upright.

You can improve your stability and balance through core exercises that strengthen these muscles at the center of your body. A strong core helps combat poor posture and low-back pain. It also helps prevent falls, especially in older adults.

BEGINNING WITH A LOT TO LOSE

- A good place to start is when your muscles are warm. Try doing a few stretches in the tub or after a hot shower. The hot water increases circulation and muscle temperature enough to make muscles more pliable and receptive to stretching.

- Try a few simple stretches before getting out of bed in the morning. Reach your arms above your head and point your toes for a full-body stretch. It's a great way to start your morning.

- Do not be discouraged by a limited range of motion due to excess body fat. Keep at it. As you continue on your wellness journey, your body fat will decrease, and your flexibility will increase.

GOING THE EXTRA MILE

- Take a stretching class. Scheduling a class will help you stick with a regular stretching program.

know
the lingo!

If you are a beginner or even a veteran exerciser, fitness terms can be confusing. Even long-term exercisers may have misconceptions about exactly what some fitness terms mean. The American Council on Exercise (ACE) has provided some definitions of words and phrases you're likely to encounter. Here is an adapted list.

- **Aerobic/cardiovascular activity:** Movement that is strenuous enough to temporarily speed up your breathing and heart rate. Running, cycling, walking, swimming and dancing fall into this category.

- **Balance or base training:** Non-impact exercises that strengthen the skeletal system and core body muscles.

- **Cool down:** The less-strenuous exercise you do to let your body return to normal after the more intense part of your workout. For example, after a walk on a tread-mill, you might walk at a reduced speed and incline for several minutes until your breathing and heart rate slow down. Stretching is often part of a cool down.

- **Flexibility training, or stretching:** Movement to enhance the range of motion of joints. Age and inactivity tend to cause muscles, tendons and ligaments to shorten over time. Contrary to popular belief, however, stretching and warming up are not synonymous. In fact, stretching cold muscles and joints can make them prone to injury.

- **Maximum heart rate:** Number of beats your heart can safely take. Your maximum heart rate is used as a gauge of fitness level and is based on your age. To estimate your maximum age-related heart rate, subtract your age from 220 (a newborn's heart rate). For more information on the value of heart rate training, refer to "Monitoring Your Exercise Intensity" in *Simple Ideas for Healthy Living*.

- **Repetition, or rep:** The number of times you perform an exercise during a set. For example, a weight lifter may perform 10 reps of the biceps curl exercise in each set.

- **Set:** The repetition of the same exercise a certain number of times. For instance, a weight lifter may do 10 biceps curls, rest for a few moments and then perform another set of 10 biceps curls.

- **Strength, weight, or resistance, training:** Exercises aimed at improving the strength and function of muscles. Specific exercises are done to strengthen each muscle group. Weight lifting and exercising with stretchy resistance bands are examples of resistance training activities, as are exercises like push-ups in which you work against the weight of your own body.

- **Warm-up:** The act of preparing your body for the stress of exercise. The body can be warmed up with light-intensity aerobic movements, such as walking slowly. These movements increase blood flow, which in turn heats up muscles and joints.

my prescription for
personal fitness

For each area of fitness, decide the Frequency (how often), Intensity (how rigorous), Time (how long) and Type (what kind of exercise) you will do each week.

◆ Cardiovascular

F –

I –

T –

T –

◆ Strength Training

F –

I –

T –

T –

◆ Flexibility and Balance

F –

I –

T –

T –

◆ Lifestyle Activities

F –

I –

T –

T –

frequently asked questions about maintenance

Should I Increase My Daily Calorie Range?

Now that you've met your weight goal and are within a healthy weight range for your age and activity level, you should definitely reassess your calorie needs. Similar to eating too many calories, staying at too low a calorie range that does not meet your current needs could have several consequences, such as nutritional deficiencies, inability to participate in physical activity, moodiness and lethargy, not to mention boredom and frustration!

First, reassess your physical activity level. Are you exercising twice as much as you did when you first chose a calorie range? If so, you may need to graduate to Activity Level 2 or even Activity Level 3. Review the descriptions of each level found on page 120 to determine if you need to move over a column or two in the calorie-range table. Next, add 200 calories to both ends of your calorie range recommended for weight loss. This will put you within an appropriate range if you desire to simply maintain your healthy weight.

As always, we ask you to adjust your calories slowly and to routinely assess how you feel and if you're maintaining your goal weight. The Live It Plan has always been a personalized plan, so don't stop simply because you've reached your goal!

How Do I Avoid Slipping Back into My Old Lifestyle Routine?

We asked Karen Arnett, who lives in Martinez, Georgia, to answer this question. Karen lost 266 pounds in First Place from 1995 to 1997 and has stayed at her goal weight since that time. Here's what Karen told us:

- She continues doing everything she has learned in First Place 4 Health.

- She focuses mainly on the spiritual aspects of prayer, Bible study, and Scripture memorization.

- She reminds herself that she is accountable to God first and foremost.

- She finds continued comfort in knowing that God is always with her, that He cares about the details of her life and that He will finish His good work in her.

- She stays in touch with her feelings and emotions in order to avoid coping with food.

- She exercises six days a week.

- She still weighs and measures most of what she eats so as to stay disciplined and not overindulge.

- She maintains a healthy perspective that food is only food, and there is always tomorrow for a treat that won't healthfully fit in today's menu.

How Do I Maintain My Level of Fitness If I Sustain an Injury and Can't Exercise?

If you're injured, the first thing to do is to make eating quality foods a priority. A well-nourished body will heal faster. Also, now is the time to pay particular attention to portion sizes. In order to maintain proper weight, energy input must equal energy output. Since there will be a reduction in calories burned through physical activity, you will need to pay closer attention to portion control and not overfeed your body. As far as restrictions to physical activity are concerned, you must follow your doctor's orders. However, be sure to ask your physician what you *can* do, and commit to doing it faithfully. There may be some decrease in your fitness level; but with determination and creativity, you can remain safely active during this recovery time, and your weight can be maintained.

Do I Need to Continue Attending First Place 4 Health Meetings?

Many people at their goal weight find it helpful to stay in the program for at least two more sessions. This helps you to find an adjusted calorie range for maintenance that is right for you. Karen Arnett, the lady mentioned in the second question, said that she kept going to the next calorie level every two weeks until she stopped losing weight. Today she eats 2,000 calories per day and stays at her lifetime goal.

Another reason to continue attending meetings is to be a person of support for people coming to First Place 4 Health for the very first time. Many times new members can become overwhelmed, and having someone in the class who has been successful in reaching his or her goal weight can be a tremendous asset. It also sets a good example of being a good steward of success by investing time and energy in others.

How Do I Handle Occasional Slipups and Small Weight Gains?

Just like other aspects of life, your weight may experience minor ups and downs. The important thing is not to panic but to prevent them from getting out of control! If you find that you've gained three to five pounds above your goal weight, we encourage you to be proactive in making sure this minor weight gain does not turn into a major one! Simply begin monitoring the quality and quantity of your food intake more closely by keeping a Live It Tracker. Reread "The Nutrition Top 10" and work to incorporate those healthy behaviors back into your life. Next, assess how physically active you are and consider taking it up a notch. Review "The Fitness Top 10" as well. Remember that nutrition *combined with* physical activity is the most successful approach to efficient and effective weight loss. Also, do an emotional inventory, and consider whether or not food has become a coping mechanism or major source of comfort in your life. Work to determine the real issue at hand. Once that issue is dealt with, the symptoms of extra pounds and inches will soon go away.

Should I Continue Keeping a Live It Tracker Now That I've Reached My Goal?

Once you reach your goal weight, whether or not to continue keeping a Live It Tracker is a personal decision based on several things. The Live It Tracker is designed to help you develop an awareness of what you are eating and your level of physical activity. Awareness is a key step in establishing and maintaining good lifetime eating and exercise habits. If you have developed this skill to the point that you are now confident in keeping an accurate mental record of what you are eating and how much you're exercising on a daily basis, then you may not need to keep a Tracker. If you are not confident in this skill, it would be a good idea to keep the Tracker to prevent setbacks. It's also worth mentioning that studies show that those who keep good records of their successes are more likely to maintain those levels of success.

Now That I've Reached My Weight-Loss Goal, What Other Goals Should I Set?

Setting additional goals is one way you can ensure maintenance of what you have accomplished. It is important that you have a goal before you in each of the four areas of your life: physical, mental, emotional and spiritual. Being at a maintenance level is the perfect time to think about going the extra mile in each of these areas. A physical goal might be to train for an athletic event. A mental goal might be to memorize an entire chapter of Scripture. An emotional goal might be to invest quality time in a relationship that needs attention. A spiritual goal might be to share your faith with at least one person a week. Setting new goals is a great strategy for staying motivated and maintaining your current level of wellness (and for not slipping back into old behaviors).

Should I Become a Leader of a First Place 4 Health Group?

Investing in the success of others is always a good idea, and in fact, it is one way of being a good steward of what God has accomplished in you. If you are not confident in leading a group, you might consider co-leading, coming alongside someone else specifically, or offering prayer support for the group.

Even Though I Am Now at My Lifetime Goal Weight, I Still Have Fat on My Belly, Hips and Thighs That Cannot Be Dieted or Exercised Away. Can It Be Surgically Removed?

Excess fat around the hips, thighs and stomach can indeed be suctioned away by a technique known as suction lipectomy. The operation is expensive, and though not dangerous when skillfully performed, it does entail some risk of disappointment. If your skin does not contract sufficiently after the operation, the new contours may not please you any better than the old, and no one knows how long you will remain free of fat deposits. You should try exercise first, but if your fatty deposits prove to be irreducible even if you are at a normal weight, a lipectomy may be a safe—but costly—solution.

Now That I Have Reached My Lifetime Goal in First Place 4 Health, I Find That I Don't Know What Comes Next. I've Struggled with Weight for So Long, What Do I Do Next?

We asked this question of three First Place 4 Health members who have reached their lifetime goal. Mark Gutierrez, of Chino, California, said that he set some new fitness goals. He started jogging—something he could never have done when he was so overweight. Mark committed to run 12 races in 12 months; three 5Ks, three 10Ks, three half-marathons and three marathons. Mark was able to reach his goal and continues to set ambitious goals for the future.

Tamara Fisher has lost 140 pounds in First Place 4 Health; and her husband, Kevin, has lost 115 pounds. They are the parents of four young children and have been blessed to see changes in not only their lives but also the lives of their children. Tamara and Kevin have grown to love participating in triathlons together. They enjoy the quality time together that training and races provide; and secondary to the many healthy changes they've adopted, Tamara and Kevin say that their marriage is stronger than it has ever been.

What Are Some Pitfalls I Need to Avoid?

Now that you have reached your goal weight, we think it is important to get rid of all your "fat" clothes so that there is no thought of ever going back to where you were. You might want to keep one of your largest pair of slacks in case you are asked to tell your story and need a visual, but don't use them or any other piece of your "before" clothing as a crutch.

Also, ask God to bring friends into your life who share the same goals that you have for total health—physically, mentally, emotionally and spiritually. Proverbs 27:17 says, "As iron sharpens iron so one man sharpens another," so pray for the manifestation of relationships that will sharpen and encourage you!

Most important, continue for the rest of your life the healthy lifestyle you've adopted! Many who reach their goal feel they can relax and not be as vigilant in all four areas as they were when they were losing weight. This is a natural feeling after so much hard work, but those who have kept off their excess weight for a long time say that weight gain is inevitable without a complete lifestyle change. Thinking *This won't hurt this one time* can lead to disastrous results if continued day after day. Each one of the four areas is equally important to your total health, so work each day to keep them thriving and strong.

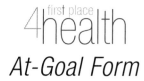

At-Goal Form

CONGRATULATIONS!
YOU HAVE REACHED YOUR LIFETIME GOAL!

When you have reached your lifetime weight-loss goal *and* maintained it for eight weeks, First Place 4 Health will recognize your accomplishments by sending you a special gift after we receive this completed form. The form must be signed by your First Place 4 Health leader.

Today's Date _____ Date of Birth _____

Name _____

Street Address _____

City, State, Zip Code _____

Home Phone _____ Email _____

First Place 4 Health Location _____

Current Leader(s) _____

Street Address _____

City, State, Zip Code _____

Beginning Date _____ Beginning Weight _____

Goal Date _____ Goal Weight _____

My life before coming to First Place 4 Health:

_____

_____

_____

The circumstances that led me to join First Place 4 Health:

_____

_____

_____

The truth I have come to understand in First Place 4 Health:

_____

_____

_____

The effects of First Place 4 Health on my life:

Physical

_____

_____

_____

Mental

_____

_____

_____

Emotional

_____

_____

_____

Spiritual

_____

_____

_____

A word of encouragement to others about my experience:

_____

_____

_____

If available, please include photos of yourself before and after your weight loss.

Please sign below if you will give First Place 4 Health permission to use this information in a future First Place 4 Health publication or website.

Signed _____ Date _____

First Place 4 Health Leader Signature _____ Date _____

Mail this form to:
First Place 4 Health
7401 Katy Freeway
Houston, TX 77024

first place 4 health recommended resources

BOOKS

Emotional Health

Allender, Dan B. *The Wounded Heart*. Colorado Springs, CO: NavPress, 1995.

Cloud, Henry, and Henry Townsend. *Boundaries*. Grand Rapids, MI: Zondervan Publishing House, 2004.

Hemfelt, Robert, Frank Minirth, and Paul Meier. *Love Is a Choice*. Nashville, TN: Thomas Nelson, 1996.

McClure, Cynthia Rowland. *The Courage to Go On: Life After Addiction*. Grand Rapids, MI: Baker Book House, 1990.

Minirth, Frank, and Paul Meier. *Love Hunger*. Grand Rapids, MI: Zondervan Publishing House, 2004.

Mitchell, William. *Winning in the Land of Giants*. Wheaton, IL: Tyndale House Publishers, 1997.

Seamands, David A. *Healing for Damaged Emotions*. Wheaton, IL: Victor Books, 1991.

Smalley, Gary, and John Trent. *The Gift of the Blessing*. Nashville, TN: Thomas Nelson, 1993.

Thurman, Chris. *The Lies We Believe*. Nashville, TN: Thomas Nelson, 2003.

Mental Health

Anderson, Neil T., and Rich Miller. *Walking in Freedom*. Ventura, CA: Regal Books, 1999.

Dobson, James. *Emotions: Can You Trust Them?* Ventura, CA: Regal Books, 2003.

Eims, Leroy. *Be the Leader You Were Meant to Be*. Wheaton, IL: Victor Books, 2002.

Hummel, Charles E. *Freedom from Tyranny of the Urgent*. Downers Grove, IL: InverVarsity Press, 1997.

Larson, Kate. *Progress, Not Perfection*. Andover, MN: Expert Publishers, Inc., 2007.

Lewis, Carole. *Choosing to Change*. Ventura, CA: Gospel Light, 2001.

———. *Stop It!* Ventura, CA: Regal Books, 2005.

———. *A Thankful Heart*. Ventura, CA: Regal Books, 2005.

Lewis, Carole, and W. Terry Whalin. *First Place*. Ventura, CA: Gospel Light, 2001.

Littauer, Florence. *Your Personality Tree*. Dallas, TX: Word Publishing, 1989.

Russel, Rex. *What the Bible Says About Healthy Living*. Ventura, CA: Gospel Light, 2006.

Swenson, Richard A. *Margin*. Colorado Springs, CO: Navpress, 2004.

———. *The Overload Syndrome*. Colorado Springs, CO: Navpress, 1999.

Wansink, Brian. *Mindless Eating: Why We Eat More Than We Think*. New York: Bantam Books, 2006.

Zigler, Zig. *See You at the Top*. Westwood, NJ: H. Revell Publishers, 2000.

———. *Top Performance*. Gretna, LA: Pelican Publishing Company, 2004.

Physical Health

American College of Sports Medicine. *ACSM Fitness Book*. Champaign, IL: Human Kinetics, 2003.

Borushek, Allan. *Calorie King, Calorie, Fat and Carbohydrate Counter*. Costa Mesa, CA: Family Health Publications, 2006.

Couey, Richard. *Building God's Temple*. Edina, MN: Burgess International Group, 1994.

Duyff, Roberta Larson. *A(merican) D(ietetic) A(ssociation) Complete Food and Nutrition Guide*. Minnetonka, MN: Chronimed Publishing, 2006.

Larson, Susie. *Balance That Works When Life Doesn't*. Eugene, OR: Harvest Publishers, 2005.

Messinger, Lisa. *Why Should I Eat Better?* Garden City Park, NY: Avery Publishing Group, 1993.

Monk, Arlene; International Diabetes Center. *Convenience Food Facts*. Minneapolis, MN: IDC Publishing, 1997.

Franz, Marion J.; International Diabetes Center. *Fast Food Facts*. Minneapolis, MN: IDC Publishing, 1998.

Swanson, Jill Krieger. *Simply Beautiful*. Minneapolis, MN: River City Press, Inc., 2005.

Zied, Elisa, and Ruth Winter. *So What Can I Eat?!: How to Make Sense of the New Dietary Guidelines for Americans and Make Them Your Own*. Hoboken, NJ: John Wiley and Sons, Inc., 2006.

Spiritual Health

Anderson, Neil T. *Living Free in Christ*. Ventura, CA: Regal Books, 1993.

———. *Victory Over the Darkness*. Ventura, CA: Regal Books, 2000.

———. *Victory Over the Darkness Study Guide*. Ventura, CA: Regal Books, 1994.

Anderson, Neil T., and Mike and Julia Quarles. *One Day at a Time*. Ventura, CA: Regal Publishers, 2000.

Beckwith, Mary, and Kathi Mills, comp. *A Moment a Day*. Ventura, CA: Regal Books, 1988.

Blackaby, Henry, and Claude King. *Experiencing God*. Nashville, TN: Broadman and Holman Publishers, 2007.

Blackaby, Henry, and Richard Skinner. *Called and Accountable*. Birmingham, AL: New Hope Publishers, 2002.

Chambers, Oswald. *My Utmost for His Highest*. Grand Rapids, MI: Discovery House Publishers, 2006.

Christianson, Evelyn. *Lord, Change Me.* Wheaton, IL: Victor Books, 1993.

Foster, Richard J. *Celebration of Discipline.* San Francisco: HarperCollins Publisher, 1988.

Hayford, Jack. *The Heart of Praise.* Ventura, CA: Regal Books, 2005.

Hill, Stephen. *Daily Awakenings.* Ventura, CA: Regal Books, 2000.

Hughes, Selwyn, and Thomas Kinkade. *Every Day Light.* Nashville, TN: Broadman and Holman Publishers, 1997.

Hull, John, and Tim Elmore. *Pivotal Praying.* Nashville, TN: Nelson Books, 2002.

Hybels, Bill. *Honest to God?* Grand Rapids, MI: Zondervan Publishing House, 1992.

———. *Too Busy Not to Pray.* Downers Grove, IL: InterVarsity Press, 1998.

Jeremiah, David. *My Heart's Desire.* Brentwood, TN: Integrity Publishers, 2004.

———. *Slaying the Giants in Your Life.* Nashville, TN: Nelson Books, 2002.

Mears, Henrietta C. *What the Bible Is All About,* visual ed. Ventura, CA: Regal Books, 2007. (Available in *KJV* and *NIV.*)

Moore, Beth. *Praying God's Word.* Nashville, TN: Broadman and Holman Publishers, 2000.

Morris, David. *A Lifestyle of Worship.* Ventura, CA: Renew, 1999.

Peterson, Eugene H. *Praying with the Psalms.* San Francisco: HarperCollins, 1993.

Phillips, Bob, and Steve Miller. *What the Bible Says About . . .* Ventura, CA: Regal Books, 2000.

Sheets, Dutch. *Watchman Prayer.* Ventura, CA: Regal Books, 2001.

Stockstill, Larry. *The One Year® Devotional.* Ventura, CA: Regal Books, 1998.

Towns, Elmer. *Biblical Meditation for Spiritual Breakthrough.* Ventura, CA: Regal Books, 1998.

———. *Praying the Lord's Prayer for Spiritual Breakthrough.* Ventura, CA: Regal Books, 1997.

Warren, Rick. *God's Power to Change Your Life.* Foothills Ranch, CA: The Encouraging Word, 2006.

COOKBOOKS

American Diabetes Association. *Brand-Name Diabetic Meals in Minutes.* Alexandria, VA: American Diabetes Association, 1997.

———. *Month of Meals #1: Classic Cooking.* Alexandria, VA: American Diabetes Association, 2002.

———. *Month of Meals #2: Ethnic Delights.* Alexandria, VA: American Diabetes, 1998.

———. *Month of Meals #3: Meals in Minutes.* Alexandria, VA: American Diabetes Association, 2002.

———. *Month of Meals #4: Old-Time Favorites.* Alexandria, VA: American Diabetes Association, 2002.

———. *Month of Meals #5: Vegetarian.* Alexandria, VA: American Diabetes Association, 2003.

———. *Snack, Munch, Nibble, Nosh Cookbook.* Alexandria, VA: American Diabetes Association, 2006.

Taste of Home Down-Home Diabetic Cookbook. Greendale, WI: Reiman Publications, L.P., 1996.

Gassenheimer, Linda. *Vegetarian Dinner in Minutes.* San Francisco: Chronicle Books, 1997.

Johnson, Holley Contri, ed. *The Best of Cooking Light.* Birmingham, AL: Oxmoore House, Inc., 2004.

Nissenberg, Sandra K., and Barbara N. Pearl. *Brown Bag Success.* Minnetonka, MN: Chronimed Publishing, 1997.

NEWSLETTERS AND MAGAZINES

First Place 4 Health Newsletter
7401 Katy Freeway, Houston, TX 77024
1-800-727-5223

The Johns Hopkins Medical Letter: *Health After 50*
University Health Publishing, 6 Trowbridge Drive, Bethel, CT 06801
1-800-829-0422

Nutrition Action Healthletter
1875 Connecticut Ave. N.W., Suite 300, Washington, DC 20009-5728

Prevention magazine
P.O. Box 7319, Red Oak, IA 51591-0319
1-800-813-8070

Tufts University Health and Nutrition Newsletter
P. O. Box 420235, Palm Coast, FL 32142-0235
1-800-274-7581

University of California, Berkeley Wellness Letter
590F University Hall, School of Public Health, UC Berkeley, Berkeley, CA 94720-7360
1-800-829-9170

University of Texas Lifetime Health Letter
P.O. Box 42034-0342
1-800-829-9177

WEBSITES

Bible Study

Bibles.net: The Internet's Number One Directory of Online Bibles and Biblical Reference
    Material. www.bibles.net
E-Sword: The Sword of the Lord with an Electronic Edge: www.e-sword.net
International Bible Society: www.ibs.org

Food Related and Dietary Analysis

Agricultural Research Service Nutrient Data Laboratory: www.nal.usda.gov/fnic/
    foodcomp/search
New American Plate, The: www.aicr.org/site/PageServer?pagename=pub_nap_index_21
Food Allergy and Anaphylaxis Network: www.foodallergy.org
Food Labeling and Nutrition: www.cfsan.fda.gov/label.html
Fruits and Veggies Matter: www.fruitsandveggiesmatter.gov
Nutrition Facts and Calorie Counter: www.nutritiondata.com
Portion Distortion Interactive Quiz: hp2010.nhlbihin.net/portion

Organizations, Professional and Nonprofit

American Cancer Society: www.cancer.org

American Council on Exercise: www.acefitness.org

American Diabetes Association: www.diabetes.org

American Dietetic Association: www.eatright.org

American Heart Association: www.americanheart.org

American Institute for Cancer Research: www.aicr.org

Center for Nutrition Policy and Promotion: www.cnpp.usda.gov

Center for Science in the Public Interest: www.cspinet.org

National Diabetes Education Program: www.ndep.nih.gov

Recipes

All Recipes: allrecipes.com

Better Recipes: www.betterrecipes.com

Delicious Decisions from the American Heart Association: www.deliciousdecisions.org

Epicurious: www.epicurious.com/recipesmenus/healthy/recipes

Food Network (TV): www.foodnetwork.com/food/lf_health

Low-Fat Recipes: www.low-fat-recipes.com

U. S. Government Information Sites

Center for Disease Control and Prevention, Fruits and Veggies Matter: www.fruitsandveggiesmatter.gov

Dietary Guidelines for Americans: www.health.gov/dietaryguidellines

HealthierUS.gov: www.healthierus.gov

MyPyramid: www.mypyramid.gov

Nutrition.gov: www.nutrition.gov

Office of Dietary Supplements: dietary-supplements.info.nih.gov

President's Council on Physical Fitness and Sports, The: www.fitness.gov

Miscellaneous

Body and Soul Ministries: www.bodyandsoul.org

First Place 4 Health: www.firstplace4health.com

Gospel Light: www.gospellight.com

Mayo Clinic Medical Information and Tools for Healthier Living: www.mayohealth.org

MyStart! (AHA physical activity program): www.americanheart.org/presenter.jhtml?identifier=3040839

Prevention magazine: www.prevention.com

Tufts University Health and Nutrition Newsletter: www.healthletter.tufts.edu

University of California, Berkeley, *Wellness Letter:* www.wellnessletter.com

contributors

Elizabeth Crews has a Master's degree in Counseling/Psychology/Family Systems Theory and is a licensed drug and alcohol counselor and educator. For 15 years, Elizabeth taught small groups and adult Sunday School classes while also serving as an elder for adult education in her local church. Currently, she is the pastor of the Westmorland Community Presbyterian Church, in Westmorland, California, and is the moderator of the Presbytery of San Diego.

Erin DuBroc is a registered and licensed dietitian who joined the staff at First Place 4 Health in January 2007. She graduated with a Bachelor's degree in Nutritional Science from Texas A&M University in 2003 and earned her Master's degree in Public Health from the University of Texas School of Public Health in Houston in 2007. Erin enjoys answering nutritional questions from First Place 4 Health members and leaders all over the world and has a passion for encouringing people to meet their nutritional goals while still having fun and savoring each bite! Erin is a native Houstonian who loves to cook eclectic cuisine, bargain shop, spend quality time with her wonderful husband, Matt, and their dog, Tobey, and host friends and family in her home.

Vicki Heath is the First Place 4 Health Networking Coordinator and has led a successful First Place 4 Health ministry in her church for 10 years. She is also a certified fitness instructor for the American Council on Exercise, Area Director for Body & Soul Ministries (a Christian aerobic ministry), and Wellness Coordinator in her church in Charleston, South Carolina. Vicki is passionate about Christ and has a desire to help others understand the value of caring for their bodies as temples of the Holy Spirit. She is a pastor's wife and mother of four.

Carole Lewis is the national director of First Place 4 Health and was a member of the original group that began in 1981 at Houston First Baptist Church. Learning how to bring balance to her life, she became a First Place 4 Health leader to motivate others to achieve this goal. Carole became the national director in 1987, and is now a popular speaker and author of 10 books. She and her husband, Johnny, have three children (one deceased) and eight grandchildren. They live in the Galveston Bay area of Texas, where their favorite pastime is sitting on their pier watching the sunset.

Cindy Schirle is a Licensed Professional Counselor Intern in Sourth Carolina and is a member of the Riverbluff Ministry Staff. She received her Master's Degree in Counseling from Montana State University and is a member of the American Association of Christian Counselors. Cindy's passion is to use God's Word to help people experience the life Christ intends for them to have.

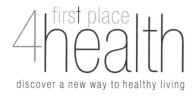

first place
4health
discover a new way to healthy living

For more information about
First Place 4 Health,
please contact:

First Place 4 Health
7401 Katy Freeway
Houston, TX 77024
1-800-72-PLACE (727-5223)

email: info@firstplace4health.com
website: www.firstplace4health.com